Fascial Stretch Therapy™

HANDSPRING
PUBLISHING

Fascial Stretch Therapy™

Ann Frederick
Chris Frederick

Forewords
Thomas W Myers
Benny F Vaughn

HANDSPRING PUBLISHING LIMITED
The Old Manse, Fountainhall,
Pencaitland, East Lothian
EH34 5EY, United Kingdom
Tel: +44 1875 341 859
Website: www.handspringpublishing.com

First published 2020 in the United Kingdom by Handspring Publishing

First edition published 2013 in the United Kingdom by Handspring Publishing
Second edition published 2020 in the United Kingdom by Handspring Publishing
Copyright © Handspring Publishing Limited 2020
Photographs and drawings copyright © Ann and Chris Frederick 2020

ISBN 978-1-912085-67-5
ISBN (Kindle eBook) 978-1-912085-68-2

British Library Cataloguing in Publication Data
A catalogue record for this book is available from the British Library

Library of Congress Cataloguing in Publication Data
A catalog record for this book is available from the Library of Congress

Notice
Neither the Publisher nor the Authors assume any responsibility for any loss or injury and/or damage to persons or property arising out of or relating to any use of the material contained in this book. It is the responsibility of the treating practitioner, relying on independent expertise and knowledge of the patient, to determine the best treatment and method of application for the patient.

Commissioning Editor Sarena Wolfaard
Copy Editor Stephanie Pickering
Project Manager Morven Dean
Design by Bruce Hogarth
Index by Aptara
Typeset by DiTech
Printed in the UK by Ashford Colour Press Ltd

The
Publisher's
policy is to use
paper manufactured
from sustainable forests

Key to Chapter 3 icons

 Synchronize your breath with your movement

 Tune your nervous system to current conditions

 Follow a logical order

 Achieve ROM gains without pain

 Stretch your fascia, not just your muscle

 Use multiple planes of movement

 Target the entire joint

 Get maximal lengthening with traction

 Facilitate body reflexes for optimal results

 Adjust stretching to present goals

Chris Frederick has been a physical therapist/physiotherapist since 1989, focusing on manual and movement therapy – particularly with integration of Fascial Stretch Therapy and ancient Taoist principles and practices. He has an extensive background in dance, both as a professional dancer of contemporary ballet, as well as being a practitioner in the specialty of dance physical therapy/physiotherapy.

Chris is also well versed in the ancient movement and healing arts of tai chi and qigong. He is a co-author with Thomas Myers of the chapter on stretching in the seminal book *Fascia: The tensional network of the human body* edited by Robert Schleip et al.

Ann Frederick is a former professional dancer, having grown up in her mother's dance studio, starting to dance at the age of four. Teaching dance students at age fourteen, she also started to do assisted stretching on individuals to improve flexibility and correct imbalances.

Over the next twenty years, Ann developed and refined her approach to assisted stretching with a practical methodology that clearly differentiated it from traditional methods. Rather than focusing on stretching isolated muscles, she became a pioneer in evolving the art and science of assessing and stretching the human fascial network.

Ann originally called her unique system of neuromyofascial manual therapy by The Frederick Method and the Stretch to Win Method. After her success working as a stretch coach for the USA Men's Olympic Wrestling Team of 1996, she grew her private practice and trained staff. Besides improving the recovery and performance of professional athletes, she soon discovered that her method, now called Fascial Stretch Therapy™ (or FST), also rapidly helped clients of all ages with a variety of chronic, unresponsive pain conditions, functional imbalances and other common neuromusculoskeletal disorders.

The Fredericks are both certified by Thomas Myers in Anatomy Trains® Structural Integration and are the authors of the popular book Stretch to Win. Ann and Chris directed their own highly successful center for FST, physical therapy/ physiotherapy, Structural Integration, chiropractic, acupuncture, sports massage and Pilates for nearly 20 years. They are now Directors of the Stretch to Win® Institute at www.stretchtowin.com, where they offer certification training workshops in FST and LifeStretch®.

Since we started writing the first edition of this book a new "stretch industry" has burgeoned to such an extent that it seems as though every month we hear about new franchises and other businesses specializing in assisted stretching.

While this confirms to us (and our students) that we have been in the right "business" all these years, this trend has also disturbingly revealed what is lacking. No prerequisites and as little as four hours of training to be a "stretcher" or "stretch technician" is all that it takes to apply for a minimum wage job at one of the many businesses for stretch services. Definitive assessments with specific assisted stretching targeted for the individual are not offered in the cookie-cutter protocols that limit the session to 10 or so of the same exact stretches every session. And home stretch programs are also commonly missing, so the client becomes dependent on the services provided.

We pride ourselves on employing what others now call the "gold standard" of assisted stretch training for the professional at the Stretch to Win® Institute. Our technique, Fascial Stretch Therapy™, has over two decades of practice-based evidence and literally thousands of clients as well as student testimonials. In this new edition of our book, we introduce new research into the science of stretching as well as our own evidence-based study that we presented at the Fascia Research Congress in 2018.

The original passion that gave birth to our book still lights each and every one of our days – that is, to help give hope and a better quality of life to as many people as possible. This extends well beyond clients to our students, who can now offer new services, extend their own careers, and significantly increase their income and quality of life doing what they really love, namely using FST to make a positive difference in people's lives. Catalyzed by us and now greatly expanded by our students, our dream has come true and is exponentially growing with each of our graduating classes.

If you are a practitioner who enjoys using your heart and your hands to make people feel and function better, then there is a reason why you hold this book in your hands. And when you're ready to receive the genuine "FST experience", we encourage you to join us while we're "still kicking" for a truly life transforming event at our Stretch to Win Institute.

Ann Frederick
Chris Frederick
Tempe, AZ, USA
December 2019

Note
Please note that the term Fascial Stretch Therapy™ is in transition and will eventually be re-branded as Frederick Stretch Technique®. Meanwhile both terms will be in use, while the acronym FST will remain the same.

It is a pleasure to see many years of work by my friends Chris and Ann Frederick synthesized into the book you hold in your hands. Of course it is personally gratifying to see the Anatomy Trains map applied in a new and practical way, but I hasten to add that the Fascial Stretch Therapy methodology is all their own.

FST is truly a team effort. Chris's conceptual ingenuity and physiotherapy background blend seamlessly with Ann's intuitively sure feel and "get 'er done" attitude. Their partnership and dedication to what works has led to a series of stepped methods that allows them (and you) to make progressive and sustained changes in a wide variety of clients, students, or patients.

The academic debate about "stretching" – as Chris points out early on – is not over, and requires years of several lines of research. Whatever the outcome, you can be sure that the principles and practices laid out here will survive largely intact, for the simple reason that they work in the real world.

Forged in the blast furnace of decades of practice with some of the world's best and toughest athletes, you can rely on the tensile strength of the steel at the heart of their FST method.

This book, like its authors, is thorough and well-organized, full of humor yet serious about the goal at hand: reducing pain and getting full and efficient movement out of each and every joint. It stands on its own as a guide to acquaint the practitioner with every aspect of the method and call you to your highest and most attentive work. But I hope it will also serve to bring more professionals to their trainings, where the details of their handling skills can be passed kinesthetically – always the best way to obtain a new manual skill. Meanwhile, this book serves as well as any two-dimensional object can in bringing their four-dimensional work to life.

Tom Myers
Walpole, Maine, USA
March 2014

When I was offered the privilege of writing the Foreword for the second edition of Ann and Chris Frederick's book on assisted stretching, Fascial Stretch Therapy, I immediately had wonderful memories of meeting them for the first time after they had been hired by a Division I University championship track and field program to work with athletes who were preparing for the 2000 Summer Olympic Games in Australia.

Assisted stretching is an integral component of performance preparation and wellness care. Fascial Stretch Therapy (FST) will ensure optimal progression from strength training, skill training, and, finally, during competition. Since 1975 I have provided care for active adults involved in a lifestyle of sport and athletic activities. Assisted stretching has always been a part of my success with clients. I have been a member of sports medicine care with four USA Olympic track and field teams and six World Championship teams.

Ann and Chris Frederick have expanded and improved their approach through specificity in assisted stretching to create a customized experience that addresses the primary concerns of the client. Their chapter on Assessment offers a disciplined method that effectively identifies the strengths and competencies of the client and provides direction for improvement in areas of need. Their system produces highly accurate flexibility and movement assessments.

The FST system detailed in this second edition includes updated changes to reflect the fast-moving world of soft tissue research that emphasizes the role of fascia in the human body's dance with gravity. The body is constantly seeking balance and efficiency in relationship with gravity, through its movement and muscle strength. Ann and Chris Frederick's assisted stretching model, FST, is innovative and allows the practitioner to create unique procedures based on client needs that are revealed through accurate assessment.

Strength, mobility, and flexibility give people opportunities to live a wonderful life with gravity. FST has stood the test of time because the authors and creators, Ann and Chris Frederick, are always searching for innovative ideas and research. Furthermore, they are always willing to implement new ideas and approaches to achieve optimal results. If assisted stretching is not included in your therapy and performance care, this book is a very good place to start that journey.

Benny F Vaughn LMT, BCTMB, ATC, LAT, CSCS, MTI
Fort Worth, Texas, USA
December 2019

First and foremost, we both wish to express our gratitude and heartfelt thanks to all of the students who have graduated from our FST training school, the Stretch to Win® Institute. We have learned as much from you as you have learned from us in a symbiotic, loving relationship of mutual openness, respect, safety, and care that fosters personal and professional transformation during five days of training. Since 1999, our currently certified students have used FST professionally, ethically, and responsibly to change the lives of those they touch for the better. We thank all of you for representing our work so well that FST is now recognized as the premium brand of assisted stretching in a rapidly expanding industry more interested in quantity of clients over quality of care. Thank you for your faith, loyalty, belief, and support in us through all these years. As torch bearers of our ever evolving work, we are confident that you will continue to stand out as leaders in client care and wellness, giving hope to those who were lost and about to give it up.

A very special thank you to our partner and friend, Kevin Darby, President of Stretch to Win® Canada and to all our teachers without whom it would have been impossible to reach as many students and impact their learning experience so tremendously. Your passion, knowledge, and desire to make a difference is highly valued and greatly appreciated.

Thank you to Handspring Publishing and to Sarena Wolfaard and Andrew Stevenson for taking on this project once again. It has been an honor and pure pleasure to work with the both of you and your team of talent. Many thanks also to the rest of the team including (in no particular order): project manager Morven Dean, copy editor Stephanie Pickering, Hilary Brown for marketing, and Bruce Hogarth for incredible new art and photo layouts.

From Ann: First and foremost, I need to thank God for the divine guidance and inspiration of creating this work.

Words are inadequate for all that he means to me but I would nonetheless like to thank my husband Chris. He raises the bar of expectations and standards for our work together and I am very grateful for all that he brings to our collaboration. When one is fortunate enough to share their life and dreams with a partner who truly fulfills every aspect of what a soulmate can be, one is a very lucky lady, indeed!

A special thank you to my parents who always supported and encouraged my endeavors. My mother imparted the belief that I could accomplish anything I chose, if I kept my feet firmly planted on the earth and kept my spirit "stretching" up into the heavens. She started my lifetime of movement through the study of dance at the age of four and set into motion the original inspiration for this work. She was also instrumental in developing my love of teaching very early on, as she was my teacher in so many ways.

My father gave me the invaluable mission of creating my own special niche that I was passionate about. He said that I would need to become the very best at it and never stop improving. I will forever be grateful to him for giving me the blueprint for finding true happiness and real fulfillment in my career.

Special thanks to Tim McClellan and Rich Wenner for giving me the opportunity to develop my system at Arizona State University in 1995. A heartfelt, huge thank you to Michael J. Alter, author of *Science of Flexibility*, for giving me hope and inspiration that an entire new field based on flexibility could be created.

From Chris: It is difficult to express my true gratitude to the love of my life – my wife, partner, and co-author of what has been a joy to co-produce. FST has changed my life for the better on so many fronts – personal and professional – and promises so much more for our future and all those we touch.

Thank you to my many early mentors, especially Sifu Sat Hon and Sifu Dr. Mei Chan, who were most instrumental in helping me develop intuition and awareness that guided the evolution of my unique abilities and made me who I am today. A heartfelt thanks to my mentor in manual therapy, Marika Molnar, PT, LAC, who helped me develop on levels much deeper than the physical in her magical dance physical therapy clinic. Thank you to my current teacher of all things Tao, author, poet, and artist Deng Ming-Dao for teaching, training, and guiding me with his contemporary wisdom built upon that of the ancients.

To our mentor, colleague, and friend Thomas Myers, we thank you for a friendship that gets deeper over time, despite no longer having you stay at our home for annual visits while hosting your famous dissection workshops. Your eminent work of Anatomy Trains® substantiated and gave a grand dose of credibility to the work that we had been doing with FST all along.

To Paul Standley, PhD, Dean of the University of Arizona College of Medicine, who kindly enabled us to create a research project with one of his medical students. We successfully presented this research as a poster presentation at the 2018 Fascia Research Congress. This experience has catalyzed future collaboration with Dr. Standley in helping us develop more studies about the effects of FST on the human body.

To Robert Schleip, PhD, renowned researcher of all things fascia and so much more, we thank him for giving us many opportunities to present our research as well as writings about fascial stretching in his works with other contributing writers.

To David Lesondak, Anatomy Trains® and FST practitioner and author of *Fascia: What it is and why it matters*, for being a great friend and colleague and for graciously inviting us to add our contributions to his delightful works of writing.

To the Fascia Research Congress for giving us the opportunity to present our research at the most prominently established fascia research conference available. We were honored to be accepted by the Scientific Research Committee and will be submitting more research to be published and to be presented at future conferences.

We thank all of the clients and patients who have chosen to try FST even though there is not enough scientific evidence to support it. Thousands of testimonials from over 1 million people who have now experienced FST obviously provide enough belief and faith that there is a unique alternative to opiates and other risky medications, unnecessary surgery, and living in chronic pain and disability.

And we thank the many athletes and fitness enthusiasts who spread the word about FST to their teammates and buddies, when they consistently experience rapid recovery and restoration of their athletic abilities in as little as one session with our graduates.

Section 1: Chapters 1–4

Chapter 1: The Emergence of Assisted Stretching

Things have changed a lot since we wrote the first edition of this book. The discussion about assisted (and self-) stretching has gone from one of controversy and debate to the current conversation about research outcomes showing positive benefits. Whether or not there is a correlation with that research, a very real explosion of new assisted stretching franchises and other stretch companies have opened with much excitement and are reported by an excited media on a regular basis (Fraley 2019). The good news for us is that this trend validates that we are in the right business of training future stretching practitioners. The bad news is that much assisted stretching currently being practiced is done by standard protocols without specific assessments to customize what the individual actually needs (and does not need) from assisted stretching.

This new chapter discusses a very brief history of a still expanding and evolving new industry of assisted stretching. It also covers the negative aspects of this trend, including the lack of assessments and specificity. Common stretching methods and approaches are listed so you can compare and contrast. And we discuss two new definitions of the word "fascia" that have (as of this writing) been submitted to, but not yet accepted by, the Terminologia Anatomica, which is the international standard on human anatomic terminology.

These new definitions are being promoted and hailed by scientists and clinicians, to finally satisfy what to many was a nebulous term, often carelessly used, leading to confusion and misunderstandings among professionals as well as by the public wanting to use fascial based therapies.

Chapter 2: Research and the Science of Stretching

This new chapter updates some of the highest quality evidence-based research useful to the field of assisted stretching. It includes our own research about the effects of FST on chronic, nonspecific, low back pain as well as a discussion about a recent systematic review of the acute effects of muscle stretching on physical performance range of motion, and injury incidence in healthy, active individuals.

Chapter 3: Fascial Stretch Therapy Dissected

FST is based on 10 foundational principles that are described in detail in this chapter. Since there is much practitioner–client movement, the choreography required to successfully perform FST and guidelines for best client outcomes are outlined in these principles. For example: synchronizing breathing with movement, tuning the nervous system to the needs of the client, following a logical anatomical order, achieving range of motion gains without pain, mobilizing before stretching, stretching neuromyofascia not just muscle, using multiple planes of movement, targeting the entire joint, getting maximal lengthening with traction, facilitating neurological reflexes for optimal results, and adjusting stretching to individual client goals and requirements.

Finally, contraindications and indications for FST are listed along with new updates to reflect current understandings (for example, about Golgi tendon organs) with supporting references.

Chapter 4: Assessment

The information in this important chapter is based on, and supported by, the thousands of clients that have been evaluated and treated over the 20 years we have operated our FST clinic. It is also based on feedback from the thousands of professionals we trained that are now using FST assessment and treatment methods.

The topic of assessment in manual therapy is a complex and even controversial one as different groups now polarize themselves by siding only with evidence-based peers and training. We take a more balanced approach, accepting the need for ongoing evidence in research but also acknowledging the value and benefits of disciplined clinical experience.

To make this topic initially more easily accessible, manual assessment techniques are conveniently grouped as SSS – Stretching, Shortening or Stabilizing regions for rapid feedback of efficacy and direction in treatment. Assessment theory is progressed with SITTT (Scan, Identify, Treat, Test, Treat again), which introduces a quick method to derive a differential working diagnosis and subsequent treatment. This method will save you time when forming a working hypothesis that will quickly be proven or disproven so that you will have enough time to develop other hypotheses that you can test for efficacy, all within a single session. The flow from global to local and static to dynamic assessments and treatments will logically progress through posture, myofascia, joint, and nerve protocols. This chapter also covers functional, weight bearing positions of assessments and quick tests of mini-treatments to table-based, more specific assessments and treatments.

Finally, the material in this section has been updated from the first edition with new information and references.

Section 2: Chapters 5 and 6

Chapters 5 and 6: FST – Lower Body and Upper Body Techniques

The great majority of all photographs and artwork are new in this section along with new titles to reflect the change in nomenclature from the use of the term "fascial line(s)" to "fascial net(s)".

These last two chapters of the book are the most practical in the sense that the foundation of the training is provided in a detailed, step-by-step method. You will have the flexibility to design a session based on your client's needs. Some examples follow to give you an idea of the wide spectrum of outcomes that FST addresses, that is: physical, mental, emotional, and even spiritual:

- provides full body therapy
- joint, nerve, and myofascial decompression
- trigger point and tissue densification release
- balances fascial nets to achieve normal levels of elastic-stiffness
- relaxation
- decreases mental stress
- positively changes mental outlook
- improved physiology, for example, sleep, digestion, energy
- down-regulates the nervous system for post-activity restoration, regeneration, and lymph flush
- up-regulates the nervous system for pre-activity dynamic warm-up, corrective work and/or mental–emotional athletic preparation
- provides regional manual therapy to:
  - increase ROM
  - increase strength
  - improve balance
  - modulate pain

- decrease edema
- mobilize the central and/or peripheral nervous system
- improve posture
- correct structural imbalances, for example, leg length discrepancies.

The above list is not exhaustive but serves to illustrate that FST has the capacity to treat the whole person, depending on the skills and intuition of the practitioner. FST has stood the test of time and is growing exponentially with practitioners integrating it into their respective practices. We invite you to do the same.

Reference

Fraley A (2019) Massage Magazine. June 18, 2019 (https://www.massagemag.com/guide-to-assisted-stretching-techniques-117713/).

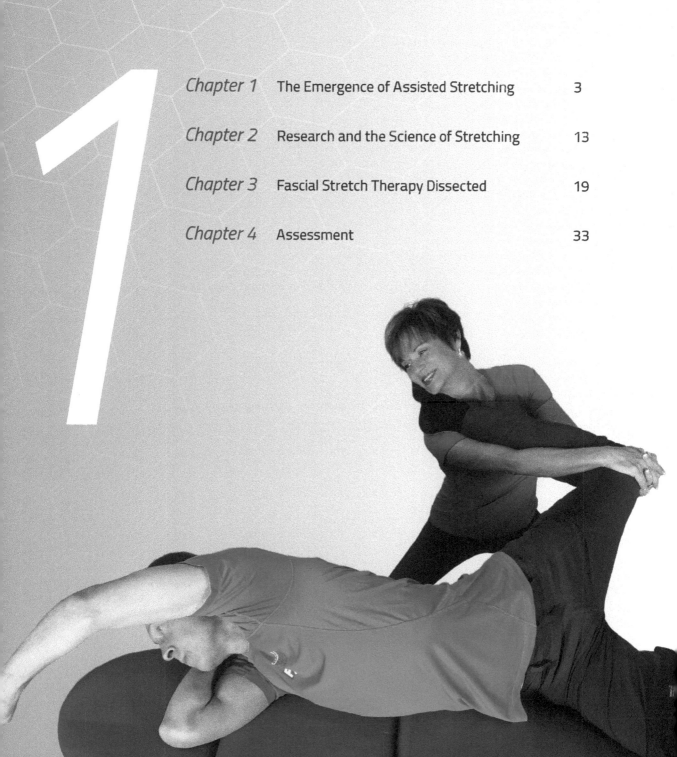

The Emergence of Assisted Stretching

In the first edition of this book Chapter 1 is titled "The Great Debate about Stretching". It covers the period from 1999, when a study that stirred an actual published debate occurred, up until 2014, when we wrote the book.

Since then, assisted stretching has had an unprecedented increase in popularity and the number of stretch boutiques and studios has expanded dramatically, both in the USA and in other countries (see, for example: https://www.nytimes.com/2017/02/01/business/smallbusiness/stretching-muscles-in-as-the-next-fitness-fad.html.

While there are no studies that the authors are aware of that describe the reason for this phenomenon, we have a theory of our own, having been in what is now a "stretch industry" since 1995. Back then, and to her knowledge, Ann Frederick's experience, over her many years spent stretching and in other areas collaborating with a multitude of clients, coaches, trainers, practitioners, and physicians, was that very few people besides herself were making a living exclusively by providing assisted stretching to help people to eliminate pain and improve performance in sports and in activities of daily living.

Many of the personal trainers and other professionals we have certified in our technique, starting in 1999, have installed massage tables for assisted stretching in fitness centers all over the USA. Being so visible in the fitness center helped market and promote stretch therapy and we have personally heard about the growing interest in this therapy and about many successes from thousands of students over many years. Entrepreneurs also started noticing the trend and investors seized an opportunity resulting in millions being invested in franchises and other start-ups that are dedicated primarily to stretching.

While there are now undoubtedly many establishments that are doing an excellent job stretching people, some achieve less than great results, reported to us by our students who have themselves been stretched elsewhere. At best, they stated, the stretching was basic and had no lasting effects. At worst, some even reported getting hurt or that "the stretch was painful." After researching a little more about what was going on, we discovered that practitioners in some stretching establishments were getting as little as four hours of "training" in how to do assisted stretching. We were also told that much of the stretching was limited to the same small number of movements regardless of the many differences present in individuals. Probably the most disturbing news was that there was no assessment or evaluation being conducted to accurately determine what the client needed (if anything) in terms of stretching or flexibility.

This book is thus even more important and relevant now, in this period of stretching popularity, since its aim is to provide clear directions, safe guidelines, and predictable outcomes with a technique that professionals can utilize with confidence. Fascial Stretch Therapy™ (FST) has stood the test of time with millions of clients, professional athletes, and sports teams all over the world and we are excited to share the basic method with you in this book.

The goal of this first chapter is to describe the main types of assisted stretching that have been around the longest (to the best our knowledge).

We will then go into more detail about what makes FST different and even unique.

Common stretching methods and approaches

We start with methods of assisted stretching only. There are many fewer of these than there are methods that either always or sometimes integrate stretching with other forms of manual therapy. Categorizing like to like makes comparisons easier to understand. Evidence from research into assisted and self-stretching is discussed in Chapter 2, while this chapter focuses on definitions, comparisons, and contrasts.

One dictionary definition of the word "technique" is "the manner and ability with which [a person] employs the technical skills of a particular field of endeavor without regard to a set of rules, theorems or protocols."

Since the word "method" or "system" refers to "a settled kind of procedure, usually according to a definite, established, logical, or systematic plan" (Dictionary.com), we believe that only the following types of assisted stretching fit into this category. The methods are listed chronologically (that is, which came first):

- Traditional assisted stretching
- Proprioceptive Neuromuscular Facilitation (PNF)
- Active Isolated Stretching (AIS)
- Fascial Stretch Therapy (FST).

Traditional assisted stretching

While stretching can be done either alone or with the assistance of another person, it is assisted stretching that is the focus of this section.

Traditional assisted stretching is a biomechanical approach to increasing flexibility. Flexibility is traditionally defined in rehabilitation, fitness, and sports as range of motion (ROM) in joints and soft tissues (Haff et al. 2016). The goal of this common type of stretching is to isolate a muscle and increase its flexibility along with the joints that the muscle may cross.

Traditional stretching commonly features:

- Isolated stretching, one muscle at a time
- No isolated stretching of joints
- Stretching to a point of mild discomfort
- Holding a stretch for 15–30 seconds.

Proprioceptive Neuromuscular Facilitation (PNF)

In contrast to traditional assisted stretching, PNF is a neurological approach to increasing flexibility. PNF should be familiar to most if not all advanced manually oriented practitioners. Please refer to the text by Voss and colleagues (1985) for more details.

While describing PNF as a stretching method only would be highly inaccurate, the stretching that is used within the entire technique has enough established, reliable, and valid data and logical application with various successful permutations that it deserves mention here. However, it must be kept in mind that stretching in original PNF was only one modality of many, used mostly for the purpose of neural stimulation to increase strength in disorders of the neuromusculoskeletal system.

The salient points about original, manually applied PNF stretching are as follows:

- The weak agonist needing strengthening is placed in a position of stretch to elicit the stretch reflex.
- Eliciting the stretch reflex also recruits synergists of the agonist to assist in total strengthening of the agonist pattern of movement.
- Adding specific spiral and diagonal positions to the elongated body part(s) yields better outcomes in motor

pattern recruitment (increased strength throughout more of the pattern).

- Maximal manual resistance throughout ROM is applied by the practitioner to the client.
- Maximal voluntary effort of muscle contraction by client to meet practitioner's resistance (current PNF instructors now reportedly use the word(s) "optimal" or "appropriate" resistance) (Alter 2004).
- Combinations used in stretching/ strengthening are related to primitive movement patterns, postural and righting reflexes.
- Movement combinations include isometric, concentric, and eccentric active contractions, along with passive movement.
- Inhibitory techniques used to decrease motor neuron excitability to increase joint and muscle flexibility.

Facilitated stretching is a PNF-based approach that narrows the focus to a single PNF technique, namely contract-relax-antagonist-contract (CRAC). This technique places the emphasis of stretching on the client, who, for example, contracts the hamstring first then relaxes. The client then actively contracts the antagonist (quadriceps in this example) to bring the limb further into the ROM in order to stretch the hamstrings (McAtee and Charland 2014). Regarding ROM, numerous investigators found that PNF stretch techniques produced the largest gains in range of motion as compared with other forms of stretching in their studies. Alter (2004) stated that "application of PNF principles of spiral and diagonal patterns of movement also produces superior three-dimensional functional ROM to standard static stretches." However, relatively few studies report functional or other effects of PNF stretching, and no comprehensive or meta-analytical review yet exists that evaluates the effects of PNF stretching (Behm et al. 2016).

Active Isolated Stretching (AIS)

The only system of stretching besides PNF mentioned in Alter's comprehensively researched textbook *The Science of Flexibility* is AIS. Other kinds of stretching mentioned or compared in that book appeared, according to the author, not to be part of an actual system that is organized in a particular way to define it as a unique method. Thus, the other stretches fell into a muscle-by-muscle stretch as required description that might be utilized for medical, therapeutic, or sport requirements (Alter 2004).

AIS has been likened to a "modified PNF" technique due to its close similarity to other stretching techniques that are ultimately just variations of PNF techniques, if only the two-second protocol is removed (Alter 2004). In that sense then, AIS can be regarded more as a neurological approach to stretching. Regarding the two-second protocol advocated in AIS, there is much controversy as to the following statement by its founder, Aaron Mattes:

> stretch the muscles ... to the degree where the myotatic (stretch) reflex is activated and move beyond to the point of light irritation. Stretch gently for one and a half to two seconds providing less than one pound of assistance, release the pressure, return to the starting position, and repeat the prescribed number of repetitions. Releasing the pressure on the tissues being stretched at the point of light irritation helps prevent the reversal contraction of the tissue triggered by the stretch reflex (Mattes 2000).

So far, no research has substantiated the precise protocol of using one to two seconds' duration for a stretch. Alter states, "The stretch reflex in the calf muscle is elicited in 30 msec (0.030 s) or three hundredths of a second. Muscles that are closer to the spinal cord, such as the hamstrings, are even faster. Two seconds is an eternity in the nervous system." Consequently, while AIS may produce positive results, it is doubtful that the stretch reflex is elicited equally in all the 600+ muscles of the body in one to two seconds. Furthermore, Alter states, "no published studies have compared the efficacy of AIS to other stretching techniques" (Alter 2004). And we have also found no published studies to date on this subject.

The "Five I's" of AIS (Mattes 2000):

1. Identify the specific muscles to be stretched.

2. Isolate the muscles to be stretched by using precise localized movements.

3. Intensify the contractile effort of the agonist muscles opposite to the antagonist muscles that are reciprocally relaxing and lengthening on the opposite side of the joint. Reciprocal innervation of the muscles to contract will also simultaneously reciprocally inhibit the opposite side muscle to relax and lengthen.

4. Innervation – reciprocal innervation (tissue signaled to contract) contracting action of a muscle or muscle group (agonist), which is neurologically encouraged to contract while the opposite side (antagonist) muscles are neurologically prepared to relax.

5. Inhibition – reciprocal inhibition reaction of a muscle or muscle group, which is neurologically signaled to relax while the opposite side (agonist) muscles receive nerve signal to contract.

While AIS bases the neurophysiology of its technique on the same principle of Sherrington's law as original PNF, it is different in that it purports to specifically localize the problem by isolating muscles and connective tissue to improve flexibility. Original PNF and FST on the other hand, first work through assessing and treating entire neuromyofascial chains before localizing.

Fascial Stretch Therapy (FST)

FST has a regional as well as a systemic neuromyofascial intention and approach to assessing and treating people. It is neurological in a broad sense in that the highest level of FST practice integrates research findings derived from high quality studies and experience, and takes it all into account along with inductive reasoning by self- and peer-reviewed, professionally published articles. Much of this comes from the most recent research and most current ideas of practice in pain modulation from concepts of neuroplasticity. It also incorporates established clinical constructs of conditions such as chronic non-specific low back pain that consider a wide range of neural networks, including those that process pain and nociception, sensorimotor function, encoding of sensory inputs, and cognitions and emotions (e.g. encoding beliefs and thoughts) (Brumagne et al. 2019).

FST is also neurological in a narrower sense, in that FST utilizes a modified form of PNF only when indicated as determined by individual assessment of the client. (For specific details about FST PNF see Chapter 3, Principle 9.)

FST also presents a myofascial science-informed intention and practice by taking research evidence into account. The following singular examples are by no means the only ones that can be provided to make that point:

- Regional interdependence (RI) model

"The underlying premise of this model is that seemingly unrelated impairments in remote anatomical regions of the body may contribute to and be associated with a client's primary report of symptoms. The clinical implication of this premise is that interventions directed at one region of the body will often have effects at remote and seeming unrelated areas" (Sueki et al. 2013).

- Myofascial chains

A systematic review of 6,589 peer-reviewed human anatomic dissection studies suggests that most skeletal muscles of the human body are directly linked by connective tissue.

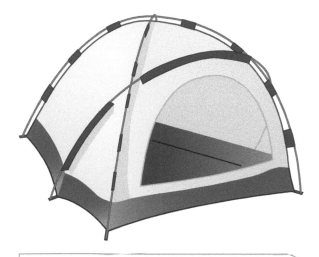

Figure 1.1 Geodesic dome tent

- Intermuscular force transmission (Wilke et al. 2016).

Systematic reviews point toward the fact that tension can be transferred between at least some of the investigated adjacent myofascial structures (Krause et al. 2016).

Finally, FST also has a systemic intent that is best described by our incorporation of the "fascial" component of neuromyofasciae. Nomenclature regarding the term "fascia" is in transition as of this writing since a satisfactory description and definition of this term has been controversial and lacking.

The Fascia Research Society (FRS) responded to this issue by establishing a "task force" – the Fascia Nomenclature Committee (FNC) – charged with improving the language relating to fascia. This is what they came up with:

Definition 1 is to be used to describe precise, tangible, dissectible, anatomical tissues that can then be used as a consistent reference for clinical and scholarly research, discussion, and study. Namely:

- "*A fascia* is a sheath, a sheet, or any other dissectible aggregations of connective tissue that forms beneath the skin to attach, enclose, and separate muscles and other internal organs."

Definition 2 is to be used to describe a broader, functional definition of the *fascial system*. It would logically relate to Definition 1 while also relating to "a network of interacting, interrelated, interdependent tissues forming a complex whole, all collaborating to perform movement" (Stecco & Schleip 2016), namely:

- "*The fascial system* consists of the three-dimensional continuum of soft,

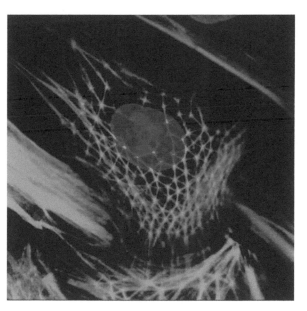

Figure 1.2 The cytoskeleton of a neonatal fibroblast stained to visualize actin microfilaments and DNA within nuclei (with permision from Dr. Emilia Entcheva)

collagen-containing, loose, and dense fibrous connective tissues that permeate the body. It incorporates elements such as adipose tissue, adventitiae and neurovascular sheaths, aponeuroses, deep and superficial fasciae, epineurium, joint capsules, ligaments, membranes, meninges, myofascial expansions, periostea, retinacula, septa, tendons, visceral fasciae, and all the intramuscular and intermuscular connective tissues including endo-/peri-/epimysium. The fascial system interpenetrates and surrounds all organs, muscles, bones, and nerve fibers, endowing the body with a functional structure, and providing an environment that enables all body systems to operate in an integrated manner."

In keeping with the clinical and scholastic spirit of the FRS and the FNC, we join them in adopting a broader functional perspective of evaluating and treating the client that "reflects developments in accrued scientific knowledge of fascia", is "accurate, taxonomically coherent, and free of ambiguity", and corresponds "to the ways fascia is diversely perceived and discussed within an emergent interdisciplinary field of fascia-relating discourse" (Adstrum et al. 2017).

While FST may be described as a neuromyofascial approach to helping restore function and reduce or eliminate pain, it is much more than that. FST is a whole body, mind, and spirit approach to optimizing flexibility. Flexibility has been newly defined by us as the ability of the body, mind, and spirit to adapt successfully to physical, mental, and emotional stress and fully recover in a time frame that meets current demands (Frederick & Frederick 2014). At a minimum, FST is a unique brand of assisted stretching that improves functional mobility, athletic performance, and modulates pain to a significant degree within as little as a one hour session. At a maximum, FST uses a unique approach that goes beyond what is commonly understood as "assisted stretching", as a means to access and then transform the body,

mind, and spirit of people to the extent that quality of life is significantly changed.

Instead of isolating muscles, FST focuses on the connective tissue called "fascia" which wraps everything under your skin down to all cells of your body, like a web, but also communicates intelligently with everything, like a computer network. Yet we also acknowledge that FST is used to thoroughly assess and treat the entire neuromyofascial web system as an all-encompassing approach to client care. (The full description of FST assessment is covered in Chapter 4 and the step-by-step basic method follows in Section 2.)

Receptors in your fascia that communicate with your brain and the rest of your nervous system along with your muscles and organs are all affected when your fascia has had surgery, has ever had an injury, or has imbalances that affect your function (Schleip 2015). That is why FST stretches your "nets", not just your muscles, and why body diagrams in this book are illustrated in this manner.

An initial FST session consists of:

- Conducting a thorough assessment in order to understand all the subjective and objective needs and goals of the client.
  - Subjective assessment determines benchmarks for non-physical factors that prevent clients from achieving a full, active, pain-free life.
  - Objective assessment determines the physical factors that can be positively changed in as little as one session, with most clients getting instant results.
- At the end of the session, mutual planning determines a reasonable time frame to achieve the client's goals based on their first session response.

FST utilizes a modified form of PNF only if and when indicated as determined by individual assessment of the client. While FST PNF is described later in detail in the practical section, we describe it here briefly.

Original PNF describes the technique called hold-relax (H-R) as active movement into the new ROM after the antagonist contracts isometrically then relaxes. In FST PNF, the client first initiates a few degrees of gentle isotonic contraction of the antagonist before it is simultaneously stopped by the practitioner to perform an immediate gentle isometric contraction of the antagonist. After a brief relaxation, the client is moved passively by the practitioner into the new ROM of the agonist up to the next barrier of motion. The sequence is then repeated. An isotonic contraction of the agonist is sometimes added for the last one or two repetitions to further increase ROM if needed.

Other than that, FST follows its original established method:

- Ten FST Principles (described in Chapter 3)
- Unique sequence of innovative movements (described in Chapters 5 and 6)
- Global neuromyofascial chain to local unit underlying approach
- Spiral, diagonal, and rotational patterns of movement
- Parameters of intensity, duration, repetition and tempo of stretch movements adjusted for the individual (in Chapter 5)
- Modulate the nervous system before you stretch any tissue.

FST commonly features:

- A total, full body stretch with no pain
- Stretching done with gentle movement, never holding a stretch
- Finesse not force method
- Expansion stretching of key joints to create more space if and where needed.

Other stretching techniques

Fascial stretching

The relatively new generic term "fascial stretching" has, in our opinion, been best defined and explained by the eminent researcher of fascia Robert Schleip, PhD (Schleip 2015). Dr. Schleip is particularly qualified to elucidate reliable and valid information on stretching fascia because of the following:

- He has conducted studies on stretching fascia.
- He does clinical assisted stretching with clients in his practice as a Rolfing body worker in the field of Structural Integration.
- He has developed the science and practical application of stretching within a detailed outline of guidelines and protocols in his book *Fascial Fitness*.

However, similar to traditional stretching, Schleip's guidelines are written more for self-stretching than assisted stretching. If we still use those guidelines, we come up with the following descriptions:

- Functional outcomes in movement, sport, and fitness are much improved when incorporating more whole body participation than isolated focus on muscles and body parts.
- Fascial stretching is described as one of the four essential elements necessary to help build, repair, and maintain fascial fitness for optimal movement.
- Stretching provides what Schleip calls a "shaping function", which basically means that it improves the mechanical properties of fascia, which includes helping muscles efficiently contract, lengthen, and expand.
- Stretching can both mentally prepare and physically warm up the entire neuromyofascial system for imminent activity as well as help cool down, repair the stress, strain, and injury from activity, and restore normal function.

Stretching Scientifically

This is an approach to increasing flexibility by way of using two traditional methods, dynamic and static stretching, and two less traditional methods, static active and isometric stretching. This method has been described as a self-stretching method, with no directions for any assisted techniques (Kurz 2015).

Resistance Stretching

While Stretching Scientifically uses isometric resistance during stretching, this method uses resistance throughout a full range of motion. While described for self-stretching as a method to gain both strength and flexibility, it is claimed that assisted resistance by another enhances those effects further (Cooley 2016). After reading books and viewing videos about Resistance Stretching, we came to the conclusion that the system is more of a training methodology than manual therapy.

Ancient stretching techniques

- **Thai massage and bodywork:** a centuries old system that, in general, uses a combination of acupressure with assisted joint mobilization and stretching, traditionally done on a floor mat. It may also be considered as an assisted yoga method.
- **Assisted yoga:** like Thai bodywork (above), assisted yoga is also centuries old. It can be applied by an instructor to improve a student's yoga postures or asanas. It can also be used therapeutically as an assisted stretching technique where stretches are either held statically or may flow from position to position.

Manual therapy techniques that integrate stretching

- **Muscle energy technique (MET):** this method purportedly originated from the osteopathic field and has since evolved into many different techniques called by the same name (Chaitow 2006). The original and

current forms of MET bear a similarity to original PNF, described above.
- **Positional release technique (PRT):** a cluster of gentle and indirect methods that are indicated for pain, inflammation, spasm, and recent trauma conditions. Included in PRT are a variety of stretch techniques that may sometimes accompany PRT when indicated (Chaitow 2007).

Summary and closing remarks

The growth of assisted stretching into an industry over the last five years has been astonishing and confirms the reasons we were one of the first to adopt it as a full service operation and create our own method and brand: that is, there is a specific need being met by assisted stretching that is not being met by other services being offered in the marketplace.

During this time of growth, we have observed at first hand, and it has also been confirmed by our hundreds of clients and thousands of students and their clients, that much of the assisted stretching now being done is: (1) missing individual functional and physical evaluations and assessments; (2) generic and not specific to the needs of the client; (3) painful; (4) produces results that are temporary. When these four points are missing from an assisted stretch session, we feel that a client is more at risk for not receiving what they need. At best, they may get a temporary benefit and, at worst, their safety is at risk, as assisted stretching can cause acute injury and/or exacerbate existing or even quiescent conditions. It is our opinion that a future practitioner of stretching must get proven training from experienced teachers in live workshop settings (not online learning). The teachers must feel the hands of each student in order for the student to get confirmation they are performing safe, effective technique. Anything less is deficient and, we consider, of an unacceptable standard. Our Stretch to Win Institute of training sets the benchmark high in meeting all those requirements and more when certifying practitioners in FST. We hope to inspire others to do the same in the name of safety and effectiveness to the public and in developing a legacy of training that meets the highest standards.

More stretching methods and techniques have been researched in the last five to ten years than at any time previously. It is encouraging to see scientific and clinical interest in this area of health and fitness. However, there is a smaller percentage of high quality research being done, along with minimal to no studies that have been conducted to substantiate the many different parameters in assisted and self-stretching that can be adjusted or designed for optimal outcomes. We discuss the research that we and others have done to advance the science of stretching in the next chapter.

References

Adstrum S, Hedley G, Schleip R, Stecco C, Yucesoy CA (2017) Defining the fascial system. Journal of Bodywork and Movement Therapies (JBMT) 21 (1) 173–177.

Alter MJ (2004) Science of Flexibility, 3rd edn. Champaign, IL: Human Kinetics.

Behm DG, Blazevich AJ, Kay AD, McHugh M (2016) Acute effects of muscle stretching on physical performance, range of motion, and injury incidence in healthy active individuals: A systematic review. Applied Physiology, Nutrition, and Metabolism 41 (1) 1–11.

Brumagne S, Diers M, Danneels L Moseley GL, Hodges PW (2019) Neuroplasticity of sensorimotor control in low back pain. Journal of Orthopaedic and Sports Physical Therapy (JOSPT) 49 (6) 402–414.

Chaitow L (2006) Muscle Energy Techniques, 3rd edn. Edinburgh: Churchill Livingstone Elsevier.

Chaitow L (2007) Positional Release Techniques, 3rd edn. Edinburgh: Churchill Livingstone Elsevier.

Cooley B (2016) Resistance flexibility 1.0: Becoming flexible in all ways. Telemachus Press, LLC.

Frederick A, Frederick C (2014) Fascial Stretch Therapy. Edinburgh: Handspring Publishing.

Haff GG, Triplett NT (eds) (2016) Essentials of strength training and conditioning, 4th edn. National Strength and Conditioning Association. Champaign, IL: Human Kinetics.

Krause F, Wilke J, Vogt L, Banzer W (2016) Intermuscular force transmission along myofascial chains: A systematic review. Journal of Anatomy 228 (6) 910–918.

Kurz T (2015) Stretching Scientifically, 4th edn. [Kindle version.] Island Pond, VT: Stadion.

McAtee RE, Charland J (2014) Facilitated Stretching, 4th edn. Champaign, IL: Human Kinetics.

Mattes AL (2000) Active Isolated Stretching: The Mattes Method. Sarasota, FL: Aaron L Mattes.

Schleip R (2015) Fascia in Sport and Movement. Edinburgh: Handspring Publishing.

Stecco C, Schleip R (2016) A fascia and the fascial system. Journal of Bodywork and Movement Therapies (JBMT) 20 (1) 139–140.

Sueki DG, Cleland JA, Wainner RS (2013) A regional interdependence model of musculoskeletal dysfunction: Research, mechanisms, and clinical implications. Journal of Manual and Manipulative Therapy 21 (2) 90–102.

Voss DE (1985) Proprioceptive Neuromuscular Facilitation, 3rd edn. Philadelphia, PA: Harper & Row.

Wilke J, Krause F, Vogt L, Banzer, W (2016) What is evidence-based about myofascial chains: A systematic review. Archives of Physical Medicine and Rehabilitation 97 (3) 454–461.

Research and the Science of Stretching

Since this book was first published, many more studies on stretching have appeared. Unfortunately, the majority of them are not in the category of what is called 'high-quality evidence' in scientific research. Examples of categories of high quality are (starting with the highest): meta-analyses, systematic reviews, and randomized controlled trials (RCTs).

Our goal in this second edition of the book is to share with the reader one method of assisted mobilization and stretching – FST – that has evolved since its founding in 1995 into what has experientially proven to be a reliable method of manual and movement therapy for thousands of practitioners (i.e. our students). It is now an essential element of preparation and recovery at the highest levels of collegiate and professional sports, in top rehabilitation clinics, and in many fitness centers. However, since this is the chapter on research, we must be transparent and state that there is currently no high-quality evidence for FST in the science literature. Recent efforts to begin changing that have started with our 2017 pilot cohort study in which we examined the clinical intervention of using FST in treating chronic nonspecific low back pain (CNS) (Ayotunde et al. 2017). The study abstract is shown in Box 2.1.

Pilot study

Box 2.1 Study abstract

Background: Numerous fascia-focused therapies are used to treat pain, most relying on direct manipulation and/or tool-mediated techniques. FST, on the other hand, uses distally applied techniques to yield both local and global desired tissue outcomes and subjective pain improvement, including those related to low back pain (LBP). We hypothesize that subjects receiving FST will have reduced nonspecific LBP and enhanced activities of daily living (ADL) scores.

Methods: Eleven subjects who met study criteria (7F, 4M; Age 22-32 y/o) underwent 1 (N=11), 2 (N=7), or 3 (N=5) successive FST treatments (Tx in table below), which consisted of 30 minutes of 3-strap stabilization-mediated body stretch (8 per side). Subjects had pain and ADL scores (Bathing: BAT; Car egress/ingress: CEI; Toilet use: TOI; Forward bending: FOB; Dressing: DRE) measured pre- and 1- and 3-day post-FST. We used a linear mixed effects model to ascertain the relative % change in scores over time using the pretreatment time point as the reference group. All p-values were 2-sided and $p < 0.05$ was considered statistically significant.

Results: Statistically significant improvements in pain and ADL scores (*) were found at the time points shown in the table:

SCORE	1 Tx; 1 day post	1 Tx; 3 day post	2 Tx; 1 day post	2 Tx; 3 day post	3 Tx; 1 day post	3 Tx; 3 day post
PAIN	*	*		*	*	
BAT				*		
CEI	*	*	*	*	*	*
TOI						
FOB	*	*	*	*	*	*
DRE	*			*		*	*

Score improvements noted in the table ranged between 31% and 57% compared to pretreatment time point.

Conclusion: This pilot study shows that both single as well as multiple, successive 30 minute FST treatments improve pain and ADL scores, with the highest improvements seen in pain and FOB. Future studies will determine optimal treatment

frequency and measure additional variables aimed at mechanistic understanding
of treatment effects. [All subjects were consented as part of a UA approved IRB.]

Limitations of study: The following factors limit our ability to make definitive conclusions:

- Low sample size of pilot study
- Lack of a no-treatment group
- Treatment was limited to only one 30-minute session on any given day.

Future studies

- Include a no-treatment group
- Increase sample size
- Determine optimal treatment frequency comparing treatment once, twice, and three times per week.

One important takeaway from this study is that it confirmed what we have already known anecdotally for two decades, namely that FST can significantly reduce pain in as little as one 30-minute session. More studies are in the planning stage for the near future.

If we discuss just those studies that are in the 'high-quality' category, the choices are few and the practical applications of favorable outcomes are severely limited. It has been well known for at least the last 10 years that there have been a multitude of studies comparing a variety of set parameters that have established poor outcomes when static stretching is done up to an hour before athletic activity requiring power or strength. Outcomes from reviews of systematic studies on whether stretching prevented injuries were also poor at that time (Frederick & Frederick 2014). That is the main reason why the majority of collegiate and professional sports teams have adopted dynamic stretching programs even before enough research studies demonstrated favorable outcomes.

In keeping with the goal of this book, the rest of this chapter will be limited to briefly discussing a few

high-quality representative studies that present relevant research as well as indicating where there is the need for further investigation. We hope that this will suffice as a 'micro' supplement to the volume of less high-quality studies currently available and that practitioners will be a bit more informed about what techniques or methods may be implemented with their clients for optimal outcomes.

An analysis of the current literature on the acute effects of dynamic stretching (DS) determined that "there is a substantial amount of evidence pointing out the positive effects on range of motion (ROM) and subsequent performance" as determined by the measured production of force, power, sprint and jump (Opplert & Babault 2018). After years of debate about whether stretching was even appropriate for athletes to engage in, growing numbers of studies were finally pointing to the benefits. DS (aka dynamic mobilization) is now considered an essential element of athletic preparation, despite a recent systematic review finding minimal evidence presented as to how DS actually affects the neuromuscular system (Behm et al. 2016).

Despite substantial amounts of evidence favoring individual and group dynamic stretching, the previously noted analysis also found numerous studies reporting no alteration or even performance impairment. Possible mitigating factors such as stretch duration, amplitude, or velocity were highlighted but we think that it is not too far a reach to extrapolate that other additional factors such as stretch intensity, frequency, and tempo may also be relevant factors in addition to others not discussed.

A recent collaboration between top stretching researchers produced a systematic review summarizing the results of the high-quality RCTs published to date (Behm et al. 2016). This review produced a summary of stretching outcomes that provides a comprehensive impression of where the science of acute, pre-activity self-stretching may be today.

Acute effects of muscle stretching on physical performance range of motion, and injury incidence in healthy active individuals: a systematic review

In this review (Behm et al. 2016), "an overview of the literature was performed citing the effects of pre activity stretching on physical performance, injury risk, and ROM, as well as the physiological mechanisms, with the objective of investigating, analyzing, and interpreting the acute physical responses to a variety of stretching techniques to provide clarity regarding the impact on performance, ROM, and injury" (Behm et al. 2016).

Limitations described by the authors that were encountered when reviewing the literature included "issues related to internal validity (i.e. bias caused by expectancy effects) and external validity (i.e. stretch durations and warm-up components, description detail of stretches, reporting bias against non-significant results)."

Based on this systematic review, the authors produced a position statement for the Canadian Society for Exercise Physiology that we now summarize with a bit of paraphrasing (Behm et al. 2016):

Summary

Pre-activity muscle stretching (done by solitary individuals to themselves or in a group) in some form appears to be of greater benefit than deficit (in terms of performance, ROM, and injury outcomes) but the type of stretching chosen and the make-up of the stretch routine will depend on the context within which it is used. The following contexts were enumerated in the position statement, followed by some thoughts of our own:

1. *Regarding stretch duration*: static stretch (SS) and proprioceptive neuromuscular facilitation (PNF) stretching >60 seconds

total per individual muscle are not recommended immediately before training or competition unless one is willing to sacrifice optimum physical performance for a decreased risk of specific muscle injury and/or a specific need for increased ROM.

Although individual circumstances will abound, we find this conclusion useful mostly for those engaged in rehabilitation to full function that want to progress at a pace that reduces risk for re-injury while also reducing other risks, e.g. disorganized, densified, or immobile scar tissue formation. As a single parameter, all of the professional colleagues that we interact with who work with athletes avoid both SS and PNF >60 seconds per muscle and instead use DS for all pre-activity. In addition to supervised or self-guided DS, our own graduates also use a functional tempo based version of assisted FST called the Fast StretchWave™ for an individualized approach to pre-activity preparation (discussed in Chapter 3, Principle 1).

2. *Regarding injury*: injury reduction appears to require more than 5 minutes of total stretching of multiple task-related muscle groups. However, when an optimal pre-event warm-up with an appropriate duration of stretching is completed (i.e. initial aerobic activity, stretching component, task- or activity-specific dynamic activities) the benefits of SS and PNF stretching for increasing ROM and reducing muscle injury risk at least balance, or may outweigh, any possible cost of performance decrements.

Some of our thoughts:

- This statement confirms what is commonly practiced today in sport training, i.e. pre-activity self-stretching with best outcomes for performance is dynamic or DS. However, if an individual is engaged in rehabilitation in order to return to sport activity, the guidelines indicate that if the person has decreased ROM or is recovering from a muscle injury, then an SS and/or PNF program may be indicated while DS is avoided until fully recovered. We also believe that a program can be a combination – address the target tissue that is recovering with SS or PNF first, then do DS before an activity that is paced and progressed according to the healing phase and ability of the person.

- What does "more than 5 minutes" mean, i.e. when does one draw the line after which there is no benefit?

- Even if multiple muscle groups are engaged in say a sport-specific manner, does it make a difference in what order those movements are produced and, if so, what are those movements for each sport, each team player, an individual with specific needs?

3. *Regarding muscle length position*: SS appears to enhance performance in activities performed at long muscle lengths. In this review, "five studies demonstrated marked strength loss at short muscle lengths (−10.2%), which contrasted with moderate strength gains at the longest muscle lengths tested (+2.2%)."

Since the totality of functional movement in sports entails patterns characteristic of combining concentric shortening with eccentric lengthening, and sometimes isometric positioning, a 10% loss in strength in a shortened position is hardly a reasonable trade-off for a 2% gain in a lengthened position. It is difficult for us to imagine using SS with such limited benefit.

4. *Regarding dynamic stretching*: DS may induce moderate performance enhancements and may be included in the stretching component to provide task-specific ROM increases and facilitation of dynamic performance when performed soon before an activity; however, there is no evidence as to whether it

influences injury risk. Furthermore, while the literature examining the effect of stretching on physical performance is extensive, the literature examining injury risk is much smaller, and thus more research needs to investigate the effect of muscle stretching on injury risk."

This statement indicates to us that we still do not know what precise type or manner of stretching may increase or decrease risk of injury. Therefore, more studies about this are indicated.

5. *Regarding muscle soreness*: there is conflicting evidence as to whether stretching in any form before exercise can reduce exercise-induced muscle soreness.

While delayed onset muscle soreness (DOMS) specific to weight training may be a different matter (or not), clinical experience and testimony has confirmed repeatedly, both with us and with a multitude of our students, that FST does reduce or eliminate muscle soreness depending on many factors that may be coincidental. Negative factors include: sleep deprivation, dehydration, malnutrition, chronic general low level inflammation from other causes and more.

From reviewing this systematic study as well as the author's position statement on guidelines for the Canadian Society for Exercise Physiology, we conclude that there is still insufficient tangible, concrete, or practical information to design comprehensive sport specific and athlete specific acute self stretch programs.

Assisted stretching research

Regarding assisted stretching research, we will very briefly discuss one study from 2015 (Franke et al. 2015). The authors chose to review high-quality studies from randomized controlled trials (RCTs) of "muscle energy technique" (MET) since "this treatment technique is used predominantly by osteopaths, physiotherapists and chiropractors."

This is a particularly appropriate review for us to examine, since at least one specific type of MET – called "autogenic MET" – is identical with intent if not in technique to FST. The authors initially describe MET, "which involves alternating periods of resisted muscle contractions and assisted stretching." And they state, "To date it is unclear whether MET is effective in reducing pain and improving function in people with LBP," which gave the authors good cause to review relevant studies.

The authors go on to explain that the "intervention was required to be in accordance with the definition of the isometric form of MET. This included the following:

1. diagnosis of the restricted motion of a joint or shortened muscle, and

2. positioning of the joint or muscle to engage the end range of restricted motion or stretch of muscle, and

3. voluntary gentle isometric contraction of the stretched muscle, in a direction away from the restricted range, against the resistance of the practitioner."

The authors also "only considered studies where an effect size could be assigned to the MET intervention. Four types of comparisons were possible:

1. MET plus any intervention versus that same intervention alone;

2. MET versus no treatment;

3. MET versus sham MET;

4. MET versus all other therapies."

The results of their search were that 23 studies were identified, 11 of which were excluded for a variety of reasons. Twelve studies with a total of 14 comparisons fulfilled their inclusion criteria, which included a total of 500 participants across all comparisons.

In the end, the authors concluded that

[the] quality of research related to testing the effectiveness of MET is poor. Studies are generally small and at high risk of bias due to methodological deficiencies. Studies conducted to date generally provide low-quality evidence that MET is not effective for clients with LBP. There is not sufficient evidence to reliably determine whether MET is likely to be effective in practice. Large, methodologically-sound studies are necessary to investigate this question.

In our search in scientific literature for studies on assisted stretching, MET came out on top for the highest quality and volume of studies by far, compared to any other assisted stretch methods. For the purpose of this book, we consider this discussion about research in assisted stretching sufficient to give you a somewhat informed impression of the current state of this research, which necessitates many more studies before assisted stretching may be applied to clients in an evidenced-informed manner.

It is our passion and intent to further research in this area by building on our 2017 study mentioned previously so that practitioners may have more practical evidence added to the literature that may inform their practice for greater success.

References

Ayotunde O, Standley PR, Frederick C, Kang P, Frederick A (2017) Effects of Fascial Stretch Therapy (FST) on pain index and activities of daily living (ADL) in patients with chronic non-specific low back pain (LBP) (https://cdn.ymaws.com/stretchtowin.com/resource/resmgr/STWI_Poster_Red.pdf).

Behm DG, Blazevich AJ, Kay AD, McHugh M (2016) Acute effects of muscle stretching on physical performance, range of motion, and injury incidence in healthy active individuals: A systematic review. Applied Physiology, Nutrition and Metabolism 41 (1) 1–11; supplementary data: (http://wwwnrcresearchpresscom/doi/suppl/101139/apnm-2015-0235/suppl_file/apnm-2015-0235supplhdocx).

Franke H, Fryer G, Ostelo RW, Kamper SJ (2015) Muscle energy technique for nonspecific low-back pain. Cochrane Database of Systematic Reviews 2015 Feb 27; (2) (https://wwwncbinlmnihgov/pubmed/25723574).

Frederick A, Frederick C (2014) Fascial Stretch Therapy. Edinburgh, Scotland: Handspring Publishing.

Opplert J, Babault N (2018) Acute effects of dynamic stretching on muscle flexibility and performance: An analysis of the current literature. Sports Medicine 48 (2) 299–325.

3

Fascial Stretch Therapy Dissected

Introduction

In this chapter we explain the fundamental concepts of FST. This includes a basic explanation of the system, the principles by which it is guided, and the overall philosophy of the system. Once you understand the concepts it will be easier to interpret and apply the techniques in Section 2. Lastly, indications and contraindications will be discussed.

Ten Fundamental Principles of FST

> **Ten Fundamental Principles of FST**
>
> 1. Synchronize breathing with movement
> 2. Tune nervous system to current needs
> 3. Follow a logical order
> 4. Range of motion gains without pain
> 5. Stretch neuromyofasciae, not just muscle
> 6. Use multiple planes of movement
> 7. Target the entire joint
> 8. Get maximal lengthening with traction
> 9. Facilitate body reflexes
>   for optimal results
> 10. Adjust stretching to current goals

While the following principles apply to both the client self-stretching as well as to the practitioner stretching the client, the emphasis here will be on manually applying stretching in a therapeutic manner. This will help the practitioner to better understand how FST may be successfully integrated into their practice.

The principles will often refer to "FST sessions" which are commonly anywhere from 15 to 120 minutes in length. Therefore, the Ten Principles will resonate with similar manual therapies set up to treat the whole person within the context of client-specific problems. They also apply to shorter sessions, much as a quick massage or joint manipulation to one body region works, but obviously on a more condensed level of implementation and application. We will describe the practicalities of using the Ten Principles in short and long sessions when we discuss technique in Section 2.

Finally, whenever we discuss any particular system of the body, we recognize that these systems are artificial divisions that humans use to categorize and aid learning. This division is also part of a reductionist, mechanistic, dissective tradition that is being superseded by progressive, evolving, dynamic systems theories, of which fascia science is a participant. It is in the spirit of the progressives that we discuss the following Ten Principles with an additional caveat: simply stated, we recognize that our body functions with complex communication interactions, involving many modulating feedback loops. Please always take this into account when we describe a subset of any interaction within one or more systems.

 ### *1. Synchronize breathing with movement*

The theory is that pairing breathing with specific FST movements properly (whether we are stretching, mobilizing, or resisting) helps regulate:

Chapter 3

- Client attitude to being more receptive to therapy
- The nervous system in general
- Neuromyofascial tone and tension in particular.

This is not an original theory in the field of manual medicine and therapy. Yet while we may take it for granted that cued breathing may always or often be a part of our work with clients, there is arguably more "choreography" with FST than with many other forms of manual therapy and bodywork, as we are constantly and dynamically moving together with the client in specific ways for specific reasons. The way in which we move simultaneously with the client during the session directly and indirectly affects the breathing of both participants, which then affects both persons' muscle tone and tension by way of reciprocal communicating nervous systems.

The movement

Starting with the movement, we describe the choreography of FST with a simple term: the StretchWave™. Originally inspired by the wave-like action of tidal (at rest) breathing, it also describes the synchronous movement of the practitioner moving the client's whole body (or part of it), while breathing with the client. The movement technique can be best described as an undulation that varies from micro to macro movements depending on what factors (for example, pain, osteophytes, fear, etc.) are present. The undulation may be up and down, side to side, in and out – or a combination of these movements. Movement of the practitioner is synchronous with that of the client, thus appearing to mimic what is occurring at a client's joint, muscle, nerve, or fascial meridian.

The breathing

All FST movements – passive, actively assisted, resisted – are coordinated with breathing

appropriate for the intended state of the nervous system. Slower breathing is paired with slower movements (called the Slow StretchWave) to achieve client goals of regeneration and restoration. Faster breathing is paired with faster movements (the Fast StretchWave) so the client is ready for activity right after the session (for example, at a sport event). Desired states for tissue facilitation or inhibition are partly controlled through breathing cues, as are corrections made to reduce or eliminate paradoxical, accessory or other dysfunctional breathing patterns.

Combining movement and breathing

As the FST session progresses, correct breathing synchronizes the desired movement, just as the desired movement reinforces correct breathing. Also, verbal cues become minimal to no longer necessary, as the client reflexively responds to timely, small manual cues when indicated. However, both breathing and movement are also tailored to the client's constitution and mental–emotional state.

For example, clients suffering from chronic pain and/or post-traumatic stress disorder (PTSD) are, in our experience, generally much less stretch tolerant than others. So they are moved in particular ways that nurture a slower, measured, positive response to FST. In contrast, athletes and others with a stronger constitution, are moved in more challenging ways that test all body systems for any traces of less than optimal function and performance. Thus, properly applied fascial manipulation through FST stimulates neurophysiological processes that can radically change strength, mobility, and attitude within an hour or less.

Beyond getting the client to breathe appropriately – diaphragmatic facilitation, accessory muscle inhibition, or whatever technique is used – this principle forms the foundation on which the rest of the principles are built. Once the practitioner and client learn the favored methods to modulate breathing synchronized with movement, the first, major method to regulate the entire nervous system for FST has been accomplished. If we can influence the nervous system in this manner, then we can accomplish one of the major goals of a manually oriented practitioner – to easily and effectively regulate neural and muscle tension and tone in its entirety. This leads to the next principle.

2. Tune nervous system to current needs

Continuing from Principle 1, we begin tuning a client's nervous system by pairing slower breathing with slower movements (called the Slow StretchWave) and pairing faster breathing with faster movements (called the Fast StretchWave). In this way we provide initial, general access to the parasympathetic nervous system (PNS) in the former and to the sympathetic nervous system (SNS) in the latter, to meet the needs of the moment.

Once a client's system is tuned globally then we have a simpler time tuning it locally and can selectively tune the tension and tone of specifically targeted neuromyofascial structures. For example, we can more easily access and manually adjust specific neurological structures that affect function, like particular mechanoreceptors that lie in and between fascial layers of tissue, peripheral nerve entrapments, central and peripheral nerve mobility dysfunctions, and much more.

Consider a practical example, taken from our experience: if the practitioner is at a triathlon event, the general goal of the client is to be dynamically flexible but stable and strong with all systems ready to fire. The goal is not to achieve plastic, permanent gains in ROM. Standard manual static stretching would be inappropriate yet self-dynamic stretching may be lacking in effectiveness or specificity. It has been our experience that manually performing the Fast StretchWave

(described previously) achieves client goals of feeling and being ready to compete or train. We perform a 10-minute full body FST session and the client feels strong, alert, and confident to engage in prolonged focused physical, mental, and emotional activity.

In contrast, if a client presents with a chronic pain/multiple dysfunction condition, then slower breathing and slower movements to stimulate the PNS are desired. As we know, this starts a cascade of desirable responses, high on the list being decreasing tone and tension in targeted neuromyofascial tissues for many clients. Beyond immediate treatment outcomes, we have observed that many clients in this difficult therapy category – i.e. chronic pain – report uninterrupted, normal sleep for the first time in years. We feel that this is one of the major reasons FST has rapid results in helping to break the resistant cycle of some chronic pain conditions and, as a result, helps to open the door to healing.

3. Follow a logical order

Having both had professional careers as dancers and being engaged in advanced-level athletic activities such as gymnastics and martial arts, both authors have years of practical experience in athletic self-stretching as well as professional experience in manual therapeutic stretching with a wide variety of clients.

This background of being movement professionals combined with manual therapy, rehabilitation, and personal training has assisted us in developing the following logical anatomical order when addressing the whole body or quadrants thereof:

- Start from the body center of mass (the core), i.e. lumbo-pelvic-hip region.
- Progress distally from body center by going first to shorter neuromyofascial (nerve-muscle-fascia) units or regions.
- Progress to longer neuromyofascial units.

- End with entire neuromyofascial continuities (aka "chains", "lines", "nets", or what Thomas Myers calls "myofascial meridians" or "Anatomy Trains") (Myers 2014).
- Re-assess previous local complaints, pain, or dysfunction and treat as necessary with local FST integrated with manual therapies as indicated.
- Stabilize joints that have been stretched before going weight bearing.
- The order of treatment listed above works best with the following broad client categories:
- Full body treatments or maintenance sessions
- Chronic specific pain or other complex dysfunctions
- Chronic nonspecific low back or other pain
- General complaints of spinal and/or extremity stiffness, tightness, nonspecific pain
- Post athletic training/competition recovery, regeneration, restoration
- PTSD in combination with PTSD-specific therapies.

Subacute and other conditions of shorter duration (less than three months) that are relegated to local, singular regions of the body also benefit from an approach that quickly but accurately examines and considers the problem within the context of the totality. However, this is not always practical or possible, so quicker regional approaches to assessment and treatment follow a logical anatomical order and can be found in Section 2.

 ### 4. Range of motion gains without pain

Advanced manually oriented practitioners should have the confidence and experience to work deeply when necessary, without causing more injury and slowing the healing process. Unfortunately, if a client's opinion counts for anything, stretching for most of them (whether by self or by others) has always caused pain in the past. We take the position that stretching in and of itself should not hurt and if it does, something is wrong. The following list may help point to some possible reasons why pain may be present:

- An acute tear is present and has not been addressed.
- Micro tears from another cause (such as overtraining) is now macro tearing from stretching too soon before the micro tears have healed.
- Local muscle dysfunction has not been identified and treated before stretching, for example, trigger point, scar tissue.
- Central and/or peripheral nervous system mobility dysfunction or pathology has not been ruled out.
- A hypermobile or unstable joint(s) has/have not been identified.
- Key muscle in a neuromyofascial chain has inhibition weakness and synergistic dominance of another muscle in the chain and causes it to feel tight despite chronic strain. Stretching the wrong muscle perpetuates this cycle and may contribute to future tears in the same muscle, for example, strained hamstring tears due to substituting for weak glutes inhibited by antagonist tight hip flexors.
- Faulty technique in stretching causing:
  - joint impingement, for example, bent knee glute stretch causing anterior hip impingement
  - stretch reflex
  - myofascial tear
  - neurogenic pain, paresthesias, numbness.

If these and other possible reasons are screened and ruled out then stretching to increase range of motion should not be painful.

Note, however, that a phenomenon called "stretch tolerance" or "altered stretch perception" (Magnusson et al. 2001) has laid some claim to fame as being the reason for ROM increases more than changes in extensibility of connective tissue, at least according to some studies cited throughout a scientific text on flexibility (Alter 2004). Stretch tolerance is defined by some as follows:

- A subject's perception of discomfort or pain
- Post-isometric relaxation noted in muscle energy technique (MET) or proprioceptive neuromuscular facilitation (PNF) may be the same phenomenon as the effect of lightness felt when we lift weights.
- After-effect of increased intrafusal and extrafusal stiffness, both of which may contribute to the lightness illusions caused by thixotropic changes in the muscle spindles.

While some responses to ROM increases from stretching may undoubtedly be due to stretch tolerance, others are clearly due to other reasons, one example being a capsular restriction; once removed, ROM is restored to normal.

Mobilization and TOC

We have found that there is a better response to manually stretching neuromyofasciae if we mobilize tissue first. Mobilization in this context means passively moving the torso, limb, or appendage up to, but not into, the barrier of tissue resistance. When the practitioner senses a tissue change to that of more ease, then a transition movement to that of encountering the barrier to affect it with stretching is enacted. Clients are also taught to perform self-stretching this way.

Traction-oscillation-circumduction (TOC) before and during mobilization movements are done on the client before assisted stretching for the following reasons:

- increases ROM without stretching
- increases ROM without pain

- improves tolerance to stretch
- helps tune the nervous system to desired state, i.e. PNS vs SNS
- changes tone and tension as indicated.

More details on TOC as used in assessment can be found in Chapter 4 and as used in treatment in Section 2.

 ### 5. Stretch neuromyofasciae, not just muscle

We might also re-state this principle as "Stretch all mechanoreceptors, not just spindles and GTOs." Traditional, isolated stretching that also includes traditional PNF contract-relax technique focuses on facilitating GTOs (Golgi tendon organs) and inhibiting spindles to lengthen muscle and increase joint ROM. That might make sense if the most prolific tissue in our body – fascia – had a majority of mechanoreceptors in the form of GTOs and spindles. The fact is that they only constitute about 20% of our mechanosensory system that feeds our proprioceptive loops. The remaining 80% are in the following forms:

- free nerve endings
- Ruffini corpuscles (with "spraylike" endings)
- Paciniform corpuscles (with lamellated endings).

As practitioners, if we are to have a broad and deep effect on all mechanoreceptors in order to correct, re-train or otherwise therapeutically influence kinesthesia and motor patterning, then any stretching (or other manual therapy) that focuses merely on GTOs and spindles is potentially addressing only one fifth of what needs attention. It is also important to note here that there is research to suggest that "decreases in the response amplitude of the Hoffmann and muscle stretch reflexes following a contraction of a stretched muscle are not due to the activation of Golgi tendon organs, as commonly purported, but instead may be due to presynaptic inhibition of the muscle spindle sensory signal" (Chalmers 2004). That research agrees with earlier studies cited above when "stretch tolerance" was discussed.

Other researchers support a perspective of neurological function in connective tissue, lending solid scientific support by establishing that fascia and its structures play a substantial role in the process of proprioception (Langevin 2006; Stecco & Hammer 2015). Langevin (2006) discusses convincingly that it is likely that the connective tissue continuum of fasciae and fascial structures serves as a body-wide mechanosensitive signaling system with an integrating function analogous to that of the nervous system.

This is in agreement with the principles describing any sound structure of tensegrity that, on a physical level alone, will equitably and reliably transmit and withstand all forces throughout that structure. Ingber and Wang et al.'s research confirmed that our cells are biotensegrity structures, which act directly and indirectly on cell physiological function (Ingber 1998; Wang et al. 1993). It stands to reason then that the human body architecture of hierarchy composed of cells-tissues-organs-systems would do the same and much more. The "more" part being, in this case, that the body architecture as neuro-connective tissue, transmits and receives communication from within and without the body, which helps drive all physiological processes.

Mechanoreceptor location

Some fascia researchers, such as Van der Wal, claim that mechanoreceptor location is not so important a factor in proprioceptive function as how it mechanically connects and transmits communication to other structures (2012).

So even if a mechanoreceptor is not located in a fascial structure, the fact that extrinsic force transmission can be mediated by that fascial structure means that the main stimulus for mechanosensory relay, namely deformation, can still occur. (Deformation as defined by Van der Wal is "stretch, compression, or squeeze"). If that

is true, then it follows that any manual therapy that provides therapeutic deformation to tissue may potentially reach all mechanoreceptors that are accessible by using a particular technique. The distinct advantage of the FST method is its ability to manipulate entire fascial chains (nets or continuities) simultaneously, which rapidly "clears out" much, if not most, dysfunction. Residual local recalcitrant problems may then be easily identified and addressed, without wasting time wondering whether one is working on the cause or the effect of a problem.

When the client's function on re-test has improved this suggests that all the mechanoreceptors that lie in that entire fascial net are likely to have been positively influenced by FST. Naturally, this is more efficient and rapid acting than trying to manipulate one mechanoreceptor or one muscle at a time. However, our experience shows that the downstream and upstream effects of our global approach allows easier manual adjustment of localized tissue should that still be indicated.

 ### 6. Use multiple planes of movement

When we first promoted these principles in 2003, single plane movements in stretching therapy, rehabilitation, and fitness training were still buzzing along. Today, it seems that most fields are aware of and implementing triplanar movement principles and techniques. Creative integration with the use of software and application design, clever fitness machines, assistive devices and tools has also aided trainers and practitioners in this goal.

Unfortunately, stretching has lagged behind, with many practitioners still engaging unidimensional, limited planes of movement, not to mention using the same parameters of intensity, duration, and frequency. If we take the ball and socket hip joint, for example, a circumduction movement takes the hip through the full 360 degree rotation that it is capable of, yet most stretching does not take advantage of this. Incorporating a combination of traction, oscillation, circumduction, and a large variety of movement patterns with creative use of spirals, diagonals, and rotations produces a more effective result.

Another example of using multiple planes is refining a structural correction even further, such as a leg length discrepancy (LLD). While there are a variety of non-anatomical reasons for LLD such as innominate rotations, upslips, etc., let's take a shortened quadratus lumborum muscle that sits in what Myers calls the "Lateral Fascial Line" as one scenario (2014). If one stretches it on the table in a strict coronal plane, re-checking may show what the practitioner considers an "adequate" correction. However, it is possible to take the assessment a little further and investigate what is felt when one adds a flexion component (bringing the leg off and above the table) compared to an extension component to the coronal tension test (bringing the leg below the table). One, two, or all of those specific directions or positions may be found to yield better outcomes and thus hold more promise for long-term correction than a more simple version of the test may provide.

7. Target the entire joint

As we know, the joint capsule is made up of fascia that surrounds the joint and fuses with ligaments that connect bones to each side of the joint. What we don't all know is that some short lateral rotators of the hip attach to the capsule and not to the trochanter or femur as shown in our anatomy books. We know this because we saw it in a cadaver along with many other variations of anatomy that do not fit the pictures we have in our minds from the anatomy books that we studied, rely on, and may still refer to. We'll discuss the implications of this a little later.

Our point here is that targeting the joint capsule, as in the hip, is often a major strategy in FST to restore painless function to the spine, hip, and lower quadrant, especially when the hip joint is hypomobile to long axis or longitudinal traction. Johns and Wright (1962) determined that muscles provided 41% of the total resistance to movement testing stiffness (elasticity and plasticity). In contrast, the ligaments and joint capsule contributed 47% (see Table 3.1). Consequently, the latter tissues are extremely significant in determining the ultimate ROM of a joint. It therefore makes sense to keep this structure optimally mobile.

When we say "target the entire joint" we are also describing what to use when a high velocity low amplitude (HVLA) joint manipulation or other joint capsule mobilization technique fails or works only temporarily. FST targets the entire joint with specific parameters of progressive TOC (traction-oscillation-circumduction). When indicated, we will scour the joint surfaces with compression alternating with traction that "backs into" and stretches specific, troublesome "corners" and segments of the capsule that have been ascertained to be restricting freedom of movement. When proper hip joint mobility is restored in the manner just described, a cascade of surrounding tissue release has been observed to have the following effects:

- An increased SLR of 5–20 degrees

Table 3.1 Comparison of the relative contribution of soft tissue structures to joint resistance

Structure	Resistance
Joint capsule	47%
Muscle (fascia)	41%
Tendon	10%
Skin	2%

Reprinted with permission from RJ Johns and V Wright (1962) Relative importance of various tissues in joint stiffness. Journal of Applied Physiology 17 (5) 824-828.

- Elimination of pain in back, hip, knee
- Elimination of femoral-acetabular impingement
- Correction of gait anomalies such as femoral external rotation, apparent Trendelenburg sign and more
- A 25–50% decreased soft tissue resistance to stretching of the homolateral limb and 10–25% decrease in the contralateral.

In addition to the above, we target the entire joint to achieve neurofascial effects. As we know that fascia is now considered our "organ of proprioception" (Schleip 2012; Van der Wal 2012), we can manipulate the joint capsule, ligaments, and all architecturally connected tissue by stimulating mechanoreceptors. According to Van der Wal and others, the main stimulus for such receptors is deformation (stretch, squeeze, compression) (Van der Wal, 2012). By definition, this improves the function of proprioception through systemic connections between joints, ligaments, muscles, and fascia. Proprioceptive feedback loops to the brain, vestibular labyrinth, and skin complete the kinesthetic communication system. Consequently, locomotion and all movement dependent on an optimally functioning nervous system are positively affected because total body kinesthesia has been improved. This agrees with the clinical results seen as a result of using FST (Frederick & Frederick, 2016).

 ### 8. Get maximal lengthening with traction

Ann first discovered the benefits of manual traction when she began stretching football players and wrestlers. When she leaned away while stretching a client, not only were the subjective comments more positive about how it felt but subsequent stretching to elongate tissue proved much easier. Objective tests post stretch confirmed that traction greatly improved the results of assisted stretching. It appeared that tissues under compression were causing pain, weakness, and other dysfunctions. Traction was the main key to providing relief, restoring mobility and strength, as well as improving overall proprioception.

Much later, Ann learned that "original" PNF used joint traction with intent to stimulate joint proprioception and thereby help improve function that required mobility. An opposing technique, called "approximation" (joint compression) was used to stimulate functional movements requiring weight-bearing stability.

FST PNF differs from original PNF in many major ways and we traction the joint only as a starting point, then cumulatively traction neuromyofascial tissue upstream and downstream along the meridian line, taking "detours" and intersecting with other meridians, as indicated by constant re-testing of passive, active, and resisted movements.

If we continue from the last principle ("target the entire joint"), it would be helpful to imagine again that we are performing manual therapy on a client. We have assessed that their left lateral chain of neuromyofasciae is compressed around the core/center of the body and the entire fascial net is shortened from below ("leg looks short") and from above (shoulder dropped/depressed toward hip).

If we choose as a global initial strategy to lengthen the left lateral net by decompressing from the center out, then we might perform the following stretch sequence for optimal results:

> **NOTE**
> Specific parameters have been left out to facilitate focus on the sequence and purpose of traction.

1. Traction hip in loose pack position to target hypomobile joint capsule.

2. Add hip IR to "lock" hip joint and to get selective, differentiating traction above hip joint, into innominate, quadratus lumborum, iliolumbar ligaments, and lumbar facet joints.

3. From #2, pick up contralateral leg and walk to your left and get right lateral side bend in center of the left lateral net.

4. Continue walking to left, at first keeping legs parallel, progressing to legs together then left leg crossed under right leg, then progressed toward and then finally below table to progressively increase stretch as indicated and tolerated.

5. Have client actively abduct arm to the point where the client feels an increased lateral net stretch; client may hold top of table if it improves the stretch.

6. Add right lateral side bend of head/neck, arm following to increase stretch as tolerated and indicated.

7. Flex legs and head/neck bringing arm down to front to avoid coming back through same path of movement as the stretch (avoid contracting lengthened tissue).

8. Re-assess response to treatment.

This is a good example of how maximal lengthening with traction along an entire myofascial meridian can be used to correct structure like leg length discrepancies and other coronal plane imbalances. The massive sequential decompression will improve nerve and muscle function and modulate pain caused by these factors.

Note, however, that the entire sequence just described is not static stretching; the parameters are constantly modulated to what the tissue requires at that particular moment. For example, traction-oscillation-circumduction (TOC) is performed with the intent to move or pump fluids such as blood and lymph with alternating physical or mechanical flushing, as indicated by the individual.

9. Facilitate body reflexes for optimal results

PNF was chosen and used in the original FST research in 1995 because research on stretching at that time indicated that PNF had the best outcomes for increasing ROM.

FST modified original PNF such that the contract part of the contract-relax technique for the target tissue to lengthen was greatly reduced from original parameters of 50–100% to our parameter suggestion of 5–20% of maximal contraction, depending on assessment findings. We call PNF modified for FST "FST PNF". This was discovered by a trial and error process with daily practice-based evidence. Original PNF was developed to serve the needs of a polio population that suffered denervation problems and therefore needed maximal contraction with assistance of synergists for the technique to work best. Our research indicated that far less active contraction on the part of the client was needed to produce the best outcomes. Naturally, our client population had intact and, for the most part, fully functional nervous systems, and therefore did not need more than 5–20% contraction to get post-contraction relaxation of the target tissue. See the box below for 18 ways FST PNF is different to traditional PNF stretching (some terms listed will be described later in this chapter).

18 ways that make FST-PNF different
to traditional PNF stretching

1. Traction
2. Breath guided (not time based)
3. Gentler contraction 2–20% (not 50–100%)
4. Shorter duration (3–4 seconds
   not 6–10 seconds)
5. Two types of contraction-
   concentric and isometric
6. Reps are individualized for each client
7. Traction-oscillation-circumduction
   in between reps
8. Changes the angle of tissue
   targeted for each rep
9. Flow of movement
10. Easier on both practitioner
    and client to execute
11. Use of table straps for stabilization
12. Unique sequences
13. Choreography of movements
14. Start with core of body, then
    move out to extremities
15. Unique client positioning
16. Unique practitioner positioning
17. Use of our StretchWave concept
18. Use of different tempos to guide
    nervous system response

To give you a general idea of how we adjust and modulate FST PNF to the client, we can compare stretching two very different kinds of clients: one an endurance (slow twitch) athlete and the other a power (fast twitch) athlete. For this example, we will say we are stretching for the purpose of improving results for post training recovery.

NOTE

More details are discussed in Section 2 under 'Technique'.

Endurance (so-called slow twitch) athletes:

1. Intensity: more
2. Duration: more
3. Repetition frequency: less

Power (so called fast twitch) athletes:

1. Intensity: less
2. Duration: less
3. Repetition frequency: more

While the general population may also fall into slow twitch (or type 1 muscle fiber) and fast twitch (type 2 muscle fiber) types, age, disease, pain, and many other factors are taken into consideration when adjusting parameters of resistance to improve flexibility. We therefore use the first one or two repetitions of contract-relax sequences as a test to find out what combination of intensity-duration-frequency yields the best response. The best response in a restoration stretch session is one where tissue release is felt to be optimal by the practitioner. More details about adjusting the parameters of intensity, duration, and frequency are discussed in the next principle.

 ### 10. Adjust stretching to current goals

Parameters of intensity, duration, and frequency are just the preliminary considerations when designing an appropriate FST session. However, let us start with these three parameters to get an idea of how one adjusts manual stretching to fit the client's goals with their needs.

Intensity

It goes without saying that the advanced, highly aware practitioner quickly determines the intensity, as well as all the other parameters that are required of the moment. With professional athletes, you usually get only one chance to prove your effectiveness as a practitioner, as they are experienced, demanding clients. Thus, when we teach FST we warn our students: "NEVER stretch beyond where your gut tells you." You will get clients who, for whatever reason, will request or even demand you give them a more intense stretch. Experienced and aware practitioners know to "listen to your gut, not your client (at least in this specific instance)!"

Intensity is guided by tissue barrier feel (and of course, by your client) through the free unrestricted range of motion as a passive joint and soft tissue mobilization. Then one encounters R1, known as the first barrier of tissue resistance, that should make you stop the movement before it passes through the barrier (Maitland 1986, 1991). Tight nerves, for example, feel different than tight myofascia and have an R1 sooner in the ROM than oftentimes expected. They require a different stretch movement, with far less intensity and duration than most other non-neural tissue.

Duration

Duration is closely tied to intensity. The practitioner may experience a satisfying soft tissue release with strong or weak intensity. As long as the tissue continues to release while the stretch is performed, the same intensity can be maintained, although there are times when, if you slightly release the intensity, ROM increases anyway, thus prolonging the duration of the stretch.

In contrast, fast twitch athletes such as sprinters often respond better if you keep intensity and duration low while increasing frequency. It is as if they are literally and structurally "highly-strung" and require a slow dance with their nervous system, moving into and out of the path of movement intent before increasing ROM.

Frequency

Repetition of a stretch sequence does not follow a strict protocol of, for example, three reps per stretch. Rather, it is married to intensity and duration and follows what the tissue needs. Again, the experienced practitioner knows exactly what this means but it is worth reading this section as performing FST is different, which will become apparent if you practice this on enough clients.

When we worked with Olympic level sprinters and American football players, most veterans of our work initiated their own rhythm of PNF active contractions for the FST sessions. This proved to have better outcomes than when the practitioner imposed a protocol, i.e. set number of reps, set time of duration, set resistance of intensity. What we learned from this was that when stretching clients with superbly trained nervous systems – athletes, dancers, martial artists, and people well connected with the form and function of their bodies – there is more dynamic intelligence and communication accessible to individualize treatment than a strict list of pre-determined protocols would allow. Protocols are helpful, but subservient to client needs of the moment.

Summary

We developed the Ten Principles of FST in response to our observations while performing FST daily on clients for almost 20 years. The principles are a distillation of what we consider essential in the application of FST, in order to get the best possible results, and are a fundamental aid in teaching the technique.

Indications for FST

Often reported by clients coming in to "get stretched" are subjective complaints or symptoms like "tightness" and "stiffness." Yet these comments are not very helpful to manual practitioners without them also evaluating functional movements and performing specific tests like those covered in Chapter 4: Assessment.

Athlete clients commonly told us that their coach or athletic trainer told them to get FST to improve their mobility or flexibility. Others came in because another practitioner who was treating them – for example, a physical therapist, massage therapist, or other body worker – referred them. And now our students report that some physicians are actually writing prescriptions for their patients to get FST! Apparently word is spreading about the fast-acting, long-lasting benefits of assisted stretching for many conditions.

Here is a broad list of some general conditions, along with athletic skill deficits, that we have successfully treated to alleviate or eliminate symptoms and dysfunction and improve function and quality of life:

Pain conditions

General pain etiologies successfully modulated by FST include (but are not limited to): arthrogenic; myogenic; neurogenic; psychogenic; iatrogenic; associated with other diseases (for example, cerebral palsy, multiple sclerosis, Parkinson's, degenerative joints, osteoarthritis, spinal discogenic); chronic nonspecific low back pain; total arthroplasty; cosmetic and other post-surgical scar complications; so-called "growth spurt pains" in young teens; PTSD.

Structural conditions with or without pain

- resolve leg length discrepancies of multiple etiologies
- correct lumbo-pelvic-SIJ-hip: torsions, upslips, rotations
- improve gait: increased stride length; decreased hip external rotation(s)
- improve posture: increase total body height 1–2 inches (2.5–5 cm) in adults; decreased lumbar
- hyper-lordosis and thoracic hyper-kyphosis; increased lumbar hypo-lordosis; overall improved alignment; improved scaption
- decrease pronation dysfunction.

Sports

- increase running speed
- increase vertical jump
- increase strength
- improve balance
- improve coordination
- improve flexibility.

Contraindications for FST

General contraindications to having FST performed on clients include (but are not restricted to) any physical, mental, or emotional diagnosis or condition that is: not fully healed or recovered; unstable; or not understood by their physician or other practitioner. If there is any question as to whether FST is appropriate, then the relevant healthcare practitioner should be contacted for a proper referral.

Precautions for FST

The opinion of renowned sports scientist Mel Siff, PhD, was that: "There is generally no such thing as an unsafe stretch or exercise: only an unsafe way of executing any movement for a specific individual at a specific time" (Siff 2000).

Precautions come down to the knowledge, confidence and experience of the practitioner in applying FST with integration of other techniques for best informed practice. Here is a list of a variety of factors that may restrict or impair ROM (Alter, 2004):

- Lack of elasticity of connective tissues in muscles or joints
- Skin disorders, including scleroderma or scarring from burns
- Muscle tension
- Contractures
- Reflexes
- Lack of coordination and strength in the case of active movement
- Limitations imposed by other synergistic muscles
- Paralysis
- Spasticity

- Length of ligaments and tendons
- Bone and joint structure limitations
- Gender (for example, pelvic structure)
- Hormones (for example, relaxin)
- Pregnancy (for example, sit-and-reach test)
- Body fat/obesity, for example, in sit-and-reach test it acts as a wedge between two lever arms
- Significant postural syndromes, such as scoliosis or kyphosis
- Inflammation and effusion
- Pain – stretch threshold or tolerance
- Fear
- Immobilization in a cast or splint
- The presence of any simultaneous movement in another direction
- Body mass – large biceps or quadriceps limits flexion
- Temperature – decreased elasticity with cold
- Age (for example, increased collagen deposition)
- Ethnic origin
- Training (for example, DOMS or overtraining makes one tighter, stiffer)
- Circadian variations (time of day)
- Personal activity patterns (for example, poor posture when sitting)
- Vocation – sitting all day versus standing all day
- Medications
- A full bladder
- Warm-up

In general, to increase flexibility at joints, muscles, or fascia, stretching alone or integrated with other modalities must do at least one, if not all, of the four things below (when appropriate):

1. Increase the extensibility of connective tissues in muscles or joints.

2. Reduce muscular tension and thus produce relaxation.

3. Increase the coordination of the body segments and the strength of the agonistic muscle group.

4. Reduce inflammation, effusion, and pain.

However, there may be cases where big, red flags warn you against increasing ROM, whether by stretching or other means. A whiplash injury comes to mind, where the muscles in spasm around it are actually stabilizing an unidentified dens (C2) fracture. When you can't do anything to release neuromyofascia, there may be a very good reason not to go any further and consider referring to the appropriate professional. In the previously mentioned case of whiplash, for example, an open mouth X-ray should be immediately ordered and a fracture and/or sprain ruled out before having the client return to see you.

The caveat "when appropriate" is determined by the stretching technique employed. Loss of motion because of abnormal bone and joint structure is also beyond the scope of any stretching procedure.

Summary

Between and perhaps beyond a strict list of indications and contraindications is a large gray zone where there is not much evidence, either scientific or anecdotal, that can give assured guidance as to whether FST (or anything else for that matter) will work in particular client cases.

However, if all who work directly on people believe in and work by the principle "Above all do no harm," then sufficient experience and seasoned intuition will serve you well, as it has the authors and numerous others. That is to say, after taking a thorough interview with the client and screening for any red flags; after performing a comprehensive evaluation; after getting the approval (if need be) from a healthcare practitioner overseeing the care of the client; and after considering referral to another practitioner with more or other expertise in areas that the client may need, we encourage our students to try FST on even the more "challenging" clients. More often than not, the outcomes have been quite satisfying and even transforming, both for the client and the practitioner.

The following points hopefully go some way to describe some of the transformation that may occur:

- Rapport, trust, and connection make you the chosen practitioner who finally makes an impact in the function and well-being of a client. This is because the client has chosen you to be the one they completely open up to physically, mentally, emotionally, and spiritually.

- When the client chooses you to be the key practitioner in their recovery, you are obligated to complete the journey, but only if you feel capable of the commitment.

- When a relationship of this magnitude occurs, healing in the deepest, most meaningful manner is possible.

There is also much that we obviously do not know or understand that may aid or complement these processes. High-quality evidence from research about which practical techniques may be applied – and when – is greatly lacking. The point to be made here is that FST used appropriately as outlined previously is often the tipping point for our clients and appears to stimulate and complement the natural ability of the body to heal itself. We invite you to apply the principles and techniques in this book and experience the possibilities for yourself and your clients.

References

Alter MJ (2004) Science of Flexibility, 3rd edn. Champaign, IL: Human Kinetics.

Chalmers G (2004) Re-examination of the possible role of Golgi tendon organ and muscle spindle reflexes in proprioceptive neuromuscular facilitation muscle stretching. Sports Biomechanics 3 (1) 159–183.

Frederick A, Frederick C (2016) Stretch to Win. Champaign, IL: Human Kinetics.

Ingber DE (1998) Architecture of life. Scientific American. [Online] (http://time.arts.ucla.edu/Talks/Barcelona/Arch_Life.htm) [accessed 5 November 2013].

Johns RJ, Wright V (1962) Relative importance of various tissues in joint stiffness. Journal of Applied Physiology 17 (5) 824–828.

Langevin HH (2006) Connective tissue: A body-wide signaling network? Medical Hypotheses 66 (6) 1074–1077.

Magnusson SP, Simonsen EB, Aagaard P, Boesen J, Johannsen F, Kjaer M (2001) Determinants of musculoskeletal flexibility: Viscoelastic properties, cross-sectional area, EMG and stretch tolerance. Scandinavian Journal of Medicine and Science in Sport 7 (4) 195–202.

Maitland GD (1986) Vertebral Manipulation, 5th edn. London: Butterworth-Heinemann.

Maitland GD (1991) Peripheral Manipulation, 3rd edn. London: Butterworth-Heinemann.

Myers TW (2014) Anatomy Trains: Myofascial meridians for manual and movement therapists, 3rd edn. Edinburgh: Churchill Livingstone Elsevier.

Schleip R (2012) Fascia as an organ of communication. In: Schleip R (ed.) The Tensional Network of the Human Body. Edinburgh: Elsevier, 77–79.

Siff MC (2000) Supertraining. Denver, CO: Siff.

Stecco C, Hammer W (2015) Functional Atlas of the Human Fascial System. Edinburgh: Churchill Livingstone Elsevier.

Van der Wal JC (2012) Proprioception. In: Schleip R (ed.) The Tensional Network of the Human Body. Edinburgh: Elsevier, 81–87.

Wang N, Butler JP, Ingber DE (1993) Mechanotransduction across the cell surface and through the cytoskeleton. Science 260 (5111) 1124–1127.

Introduction

The information in this chapter is supported by a clinical knowledge base of evidence in physical therapy (physiotherapy) and through the experience gained in evaluating and treating thousands of clients since we began operating our FST clinic in 1995. Our assessment takes into account and uses the now popular, evidenced-based biopsychosocial model of client care, but this chapter focuses more on the physical testing logic to get immediate outcomes (Wade & Halligan 2017). It incorporates feedback from the thousands of professionals we have trained that are using FST assessment and treatment methods.

The Subjective-Objective-Assessment-Plan (SOAP) style of note-taking is utilized for client records, a system that is prevalent and familiar in the medical, therapy, and massage community.

As any practitioner should know, the initial assessment is unarguably the most important session you can have with a client. Rehabilitation, therapy, and training depend on an accurate client history, clear tests and measurements, and some indication from the first treatment or training that the session is headed in the right direction. Reassessment within the first session will immediately indicate whether the practitioner needs to quickly adjust treatment techniques to ensure a positive outcome. Ongoing re-assessment during each session also enables the client to become aware of progress, which is extremely motivating especially if radical changes occur, as they do with FST and other effective manual therapies.

Depending on the practitioner and the client, FST assessment may include all or some of the following:

- *Subjective interview*: including but not limited to the following:
  - pain behavior over 24 hours
  - sleep pattern if known – is/are current symptom(s) related to sleep pattern?

Determine quantity/quality and its possible negative effects

  - medications and side-effects thereof, if known or suspected
  - occupation, to see if it is a contributing factor
  - relevant family history
  - special questions related to cancer, Lyme disease, etc.

It is our experience that a successful interview may provide up to 75% of the information needed to lead the rest of the assessment to an accurate diagnosis.

- *Objective tests and/or measurements* (note: most tests in manual therapy require static and/or dynamic palpation):
  - client observation including how client responds to interview, voice quality, energy level, etc.
  - functional static and dynamic movement patterns relevant to the client including but not limited to:
  - gait
  - posture

o ADLs (for example, transfers stand to sit, stand or sit to recumbent, sleeping and driving positions, etc.)

o movement pattern peculiar to the problem at hand, as well as related patterns

o AROM-PROM-RROM

o osteokinematic and arthrokinematic tests

o osseo-ligamentous integrity-stability tests

o neurological tests

– motor control of specific movement patterns

– cranial nerves

– vestibular and other balance tests

– coordination

– myotomes

– dermatomes and/or peripheral nerve sensation

– deep tendon reflexes

– central nervous system and/or peripheral nerve tension-glide-slide mobility

– visual tests

o special tests: any not specifically mentioned here when indicated for specific diagnoses

o manual therapy scans: may use all or some of the above to rule out or rule in dysfunction above and/or below the symptomatic region as a contribution to the clinical problem

o provocation tests: may use all or some of above to reproduce symptoms so as to have something tangible and relevant to re-assess and guide treatment

o therapy localization tests: a specific quick test to temporarily activate what is weak or inhibited and/or inhibit what is over facilitated.

▪ *Assessment*: summary of all the findings to provide a differential diagnosis or diagnoses.

▪ *Plan*: short- and long-term goal setting. All planning must be considered in the context of complete functional restoration for the client. That is, any gains in ROM, flexibility, or mobility are not relevant in or of itself. Rather realistic goals must be set that are based on functional return to activities that are meaningful to the client and may even depend on their biopsychosocial survival. As practitioners, we are obligated to help clients achieve full confidence in maintaining as much independence as possible for self-care and have the ability to return to personal, professional, and recreational activities that give meaning and purpose to their life.

The topic of manual therapy evaluation and assessments is complex and lengthy, worthy of its own extensive text. Therefore, this section will be restricted to what the authors have found most helpful when teaching FST to manual therapy practitioners. Nevertheless, all practitioners will still be able to easily integrate their current level of assessment skills and hopefully gain even more expertise through what follows.

Palpatory literacy

The late osteopath and author Leon Chaitow stated that skillful palpation allows for discrimination between the various states and stages of dysfunction with some degree of accuracy (Chaitow 2015). He quoted researchers Lord and Bogduk who found one study comparing manual diagnosis to the criterion standard of local anesthetic blocks, "The authors found that the sensitivity and specificity of the manual examination technique to be 100%." Chaitow goes on, "This study of the skills of one therapist's ability to localize dysfunction suggests that isolating a segment or joint that is dysfunctional is well within the potential of manual therapists, if palpation skills are adequately refined." Despite other research to the contrary, the above noted conclusion that a manual therapy practitioner can be 100% accurate in palpatory diagnosis confirms the ongoing need for highly developed levels of palpatory skill. In FST, as in some other manual therapies, palpatory skill should cover the spectrum of passive, active, and resistive dynamic motion and movements, not just stationary exploration. Precise palpatory treatment should naturally follow an accurate diagnosis in manual therapy.

As this is a book for advanced manual therapy practitioners, this section will assume many readers to have a higher level of palpatory literacy than average. After working closely with a few thousand students during FST training, it has been observed that there is a broad range of said literacy that does not correlate with the number of years of experience or with any specific profession. Therefore, some discussion about the specific skills that are needed and used in FST are warranted. The following is organized so that FST-specific skills of palpatory literacy are applied first to assessments of static conditions before movement is evaluated.

Movement vs motion quandary

In brief, there is not much standard agreement in manual therapy on how or when to use the words "movement" or "motion". One researcher who studied this conundrum decided to use the word "motion" when the subject required quantification and use the word "movement" when discussing something qualitatively (Jensenius 2011). Deemed acceptable by the authors, that is how those words will be used in this and subsequent sections.

Let's START

It is useful to think of the acronym START with FST modifications, whether the client is assessed in an upright position or on the table (adapted from Gibbons & Tehan 2016):

- **S – symptom reproduction**. Although some somatic conditions may be pain-free, pain or other reproducible sensations of dysfunction is an essential (although if not elicited, understandably not always) part of the assessment.

- **T – tissue tenderness**. Must be differentiated from pain. Besides being an obvious local sign, it may be a general sign of low to high systemic inflammation from a range of other environmental-nutritional-medical factors.

- **A – asymmetry**. The involved side must be compared to the uninvolved side so that you have a control. If both sides are involved or the other side is unavailable then the quantity and quality of training and experience will come to bear and have to guide the practitioner.

- **R – range of motion quantity and movement quality**. May be at one or more segments, entire myofascial chains or body regions. Determines if anything is hypomobile, normal, hypermobile or unstable from a tear. Also helps to determine the state of biotensegrity of the area in relation to other pertinent areas, as well as to the rest of the body, i.e. what is under excessive compression, tension or shear.

- **T – tissue texture changes**. While important to directly detect palpable changes differentiated within multiple layers, FST assesses this intrinsic state by way of its response to particular extrinsic movements. Using a table-based example, imagine making a transitional passive movement with a client's lower extremity from the sagittal plane, straight leg supine position to the externally rotated, horizontally abducted position in the coronal plane. Imagine palpably differentiating not only with your hands but also with your entire body. You should feel not just the quantity but also the specific quality of tissue movement between, say, the fascial interfaces of the middle and medial hamstring compartments along multiple angles of myofascial tension and changing axes of hip rotation.

START informs every static or dynamic, stationary or moving assessment or treatment in FST. You may question then, how is range of motion or movement assessed in, for example, a static posture evaluation? One answer is that even when a practitioner manually cues a client to make a slight postural shift to improve alignment and see whether symptoms change, there is a small active-assisted movement added to help make that shift which is then assessed along with everything else. Yet the more comprehensive point is that whether you are testing the manual response to how skin rolls or how a client makes the full body movement transition from the low to high position in a tennis serve, the quantity and quality of relevant movement is assessed concomitantly with symptom behavior changes. Most often, FST treatment will follow the assessment findings spontaneously and immediately for optimal results and best outcomes in meeting client goals.

Assessment techniques in a nutshell

Despite the complexities of assessments, offering a nutshell approach may help, especially those less familiar with manual therapy. The nutshell offered is this question: "What can be manually Stretched-Shortened-or-Stabilized (SSS) to improve symptoms and signs?" Here is a brief explanation of what a manual therapy practitioner will attempt to do during an assessment to improve signs and/or symptoms:

1. *Stretch*: lengthen/inhibit/release and/or decompress what is compressed/hypertonic/over-activated/shortened and/or tight.

2. *Shorten*: activate/stimulate/facilitate/compress/close what is excessively lengthened/inhibited/weak.

3. *Stabilize*: support what is hypermobile, unstable and/or painful concomitant with lack of or poor motor control.

When it comes to deciding what is appropriate for stretching, what needs to be stabilized and what needs to be shortened and/or strengthened during an FST session, having SSS in mind will keep the intent clear for the practitioner and the session safer and more effective for the client. Keeping an adaptable SSS protocol in mind helps you to proceed logically and simultaneously keeps you creatively engaged to assess and treat the individual, not a pre-defined or categorical condition. This will become clearer in the text that follows.

SITTT

Expanding on the assessment techniques above leads to the discussion of using SITTT or Scan-Identify-Treat-Test-Treat again. When SITTT is done properly (and with experience) it often takes only seconds to a few minutes to offer reliable and valid best treatment options. General descriptions of SITTT technique are given below – purposely in brief – as they are covered in more detail with practical applications, in the Assessment Flow section of this chapter. Specific descriptions of SITTT as applied to specific body regions and tissues under different clinical conditions will be discussed in a following section titled "Regional flow of the assessment." The following is a description of the SITTT acronym:

S – Scan the suspected region with a dominant hand in order to find the optimal location where testing a working hypothesis of treatment should start.

Technique

The practitioner's hand is applied in a light, gentle manner to exposed skin (where possible but not mandatory) in a quadrant of choice on the client's body. While it may seem logical to start at the involved quadrant that has a known problem, the actual location for optimal easing of symptoms may exist in any lower or upper body quadrant, oftentimes regardless of the diagnosis or symptoms. At this moment, thinking of fascia as a body-wide and deep web of innervated connective tissue will help you to better understand this concept. Manual scanning quickly resolves this dilemma for reasons not completely understood or researched. Practical examples follow in the Posture-Myofascia-Joint-Nerve section on p. 39

I – Identification of which fascial net(s) and/or what local tissue(s) have an easing effect on the client's problem(s) is a result of thorough scanning. Once the proper region is identified, serial mini-treatments and testing to find the best treatment response can begin.

T – Treat the local tissue or global chain within which the local tissue resides. This is a mini-treatment in the sense that the practitioner will test whether they can ease or even eliminate the client problem with a variety of manual diagnostic methods. Because it is a mini-treatment, the client may remain in any functional position for the practitioner to "quick treat." This has the added advantage of immediately testing the client's function without having to get up and down repeatedly from the table (discussed in the next "T" in SITTT).

As previously stated, in general, the goal is to stretch, shorten or stabilize local tissue regions or even entire fascial continuities. An additional technique of fascial shifting will be added and described next.

T – Test whether the quick treatment yields any positive results, such as easing of symptoms, increasing strength-ROM-flexibility, etc. Standard tests such as posture, ROM, neurological, etc., as well as testing functional dynamic positions that tend to provoke the client's problem are done to see whether the quick treatment had even a slight effect on easing the problem.

Testing examples

1. *Stretch example 1*: client's head deviates to right in active flexion and is associated with a right-sided, mid-neck pain described as a pinch or compression. Practitioner uses one or two fingers to first scan and identify the correct location. This is done by palpating skin and superficial fascia with intent to lengthen as the client repeats the same flexion movement. After testing local regions above and below the pain region, practitioner finds best response and makes a decision to stop the assessment and treat with FST to lengthen as indicated then re-assess.

   Stretch example 2: practitioner decides to continue the assessment to possibly find associative links in the fascial chain that can further ease the symptom and improve function. Manually easing tension of the right Spiral Net close to the right ASIS resulted in no pain and best response upon re-testing neck flexion. Practitioner stops assessment to treat the finding that is distal from the symptom.

2. *Shorten example*: a teenager with a history of poor posture complains of low back pain whenever she leans backwards. Practitioner thoroughly assesses many factors that may contribute to this condition, such as whether antagonists like the iliopsoas are fascially locked short, thus inhibiting the spinal extensor agonists. However, only manually assisting the soft tissue over bilateral facet joints of L5/S1 to shorten during active lumbar spine extension eases the pain.

3. *Stabilize example*: client complains of hip pain concomitant with homolateral adductor strain and contralateral thoracic strain whenever shifting to that hip or balancing on that leg. History and other tests suggest gluteus weakness and/or hip joint instability. Practitioner manually compresses the ilium, as client shifts weight to the involved side then also attempts to balance on that leg. All pain

regions are gone, balance improved. Client experiences success on hip stabilization program.

NOTE

While assessing local or regional tissues often involves applying either a manual stretch or a shortening shift to change the effects of fascial strain on signs and symptoms, a combination may also be used. For example, with the commonly seen forward head-increased thoracic kyphosis – forward shoulder syndrome – you may apply a lengthening technique to tissues anteriorly while simultaneously using a shortening technique posteriorly.

This method often works better in this particular area of the body.

T – Treat again. If only a slight improvement is noted, you must question whether the treatment was adequate, for example, was the appropriate tissue layer accessed and affected? Or you may consider starting at the beginning with a new scan to find a better location to quickly render a mini-treatment and re-test.

Two likely scenarios after re-testing

1. The test yielded positive outcomes and therefore warranted a proper set-up for a complete treatment. For example, if the quick treatment was conducted in standing, then the practitioner may want the client to recline so as to have the proper leverage and so on for a "real" treatment.

2. The test yielded no outcome or perhaps made the client's symptoms worse. Then either another, different kind of quick treatment may be tried and re-tested or the practitioner may need to start from the beginning and re-scan to find a more appropriate location.

In any event, SITTT is repeated until optimal responses to quick treatments and re-assessments determine where the primary problems are and what manual techniques best serve the condition. We will briefly review the assessment techniques used in FST that have been described: after a thorough subjective client interview, manual scanning is done to quickly identify where dysfunction in strain distribution exists in the body biotensegrity. A quick "treatment" is rendered, maintaining local or full body global change in a stretched, shortened, or stabilized position. Testing is commenced by subjective and objective analysis to see if the client feels different and if anything has changed favorably, from static postural shifts to dynamic movement improvements.

If the outcome has not changed or the client feels and/or tests worse, then it is suggested that the practitioner default to the stretch-shorten-stabilize paradigm again, occasionally even doing the opposite treatment test to that which previously had a poor or no result. Exhausting those options without satisfactory effect should lead the practitioner to reconsider if the subjective analysis was adequate, that is, as accurate and complete as possible. If so, then you must re-start the SITTT process until you locate the proper region(s).

Experience shows that assessments following these suggestions help the practitioner to arrive at a working solution faster and more accurately than not. The next section covers how to make these assessment techniques flow in a comprehensive and logical manner.

Assessment flow: global to local, static to dynamic

The following has been found to be an effective and logical means to think about and perform a manual therapy style of assessment. The goal is to discover which method of adjusting local and/

or global fascial nets (along with concomitant physiology) can ease the client's problem. Once the problem is eased then the proper treatment can commence. The flow goes from using the previously described SITTT to initially achieve global, full body subjective and objective improvements and then progresses as indicated to localize any remaining specific tissue problems.

Movement must be individually assessed, first in functional, weight-bearing and other relevant positions. This will not be exhaustively covered in this book, due to its focus on table-based FST. However, some essential movements in upright positions will be discussed in enough detail for the principles to be understood and applied in most common circumstances. Table-based assessment follows and will be the focus to facilitate a flow directly to treatment as it is most often used in FST.

The assessment flows in the following manner: Posture-Myofascia-Joint-Nerve.

Posture testing

Posture (aka body reading) examined from a fascial net perspective is an effective way to visually, manually and intellectually analyze both global and local conditions of the body. Posture should be assessed both statically and dynamically as well as under both unloaded and loaded conditions that best reflect the client's function. For example, if the client only gets shoulder pain when carrying a stack of bricks at work, then the practitioner must simulate as closely as possible the exact body positions and conditions that elicit the symptoms, for optimal and accurate re-assessments. Yet, it is also important not to overlook the classical, static standing posture assessment. It is, after all, the reference point and foundation of initiation for most movements. But instead of making the usual list of isolated regional faults, note how the body is, literally, holding up against gravity. Note more

specifically if there are dominant lines or nets of fascia revealing regions under excessive tension, compression and/or rotation. Then use SITTT and test them with meaningful movement.

Manually investigate if dysfunction resides in one or more regions, or entire connecting lines or nets then test the response to gentle corrective adjustments of the body biotensegrity. The goal is to ease the distribution of strain, reduce or eliminate pain if present and improve functional movement as rapidly and accurately as possible. Use your hands to manually shift weight-bearing, slide regional fascial planes, adjust osteokinematics and decompress the spine or a nerve (and more) in static and dynamic postural positions. Specific examples follow, where the terms used to describe significant postural findings will be tilts, bends, rotations, and shifts (defined in the accompanying box).

> **Tilts:** deviations from vertical, named from the direction in which the top of the structure moves toward
>
> **Bends:** refers to a series of tilts of the spinal vertebrae and can be anterior, posterior, right or left
>
> **Rotations:** transverse plane deviations
> Shifts: a translation between one body part and another, a misalignment of their centers of gravity (Myers 2014)

A. Static

1. **Global**: using the SITTT paradigm of assessment (described above), an effort is first made by the practitioner to get full body net changes. Despite highly individual manifestations, there are general patterns that are well recognized and familiar to manual therapy practitioners. For example, Janda's Upper and Lower Cross Syndromes correlate well with Myers's locked short-locked long body pattern involving the SFL

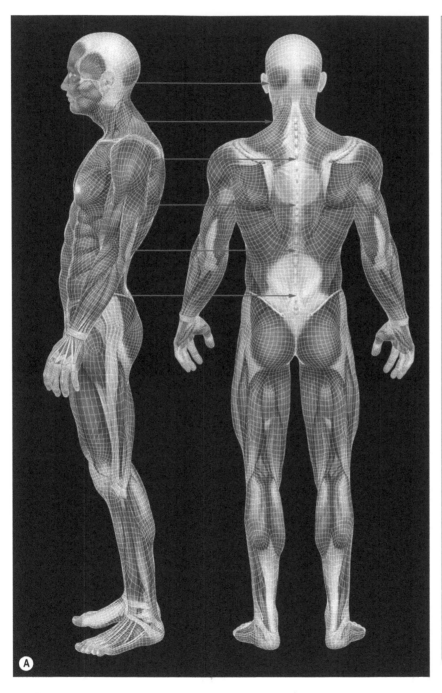

Figure 4.1 Posture deviations

(A)

(Superficial Front Line) and its response in the antagonist SBL (Superficial Back Line).

In Figure 4.1 we see the head shifted anterior, the neck tilted anterior, the thorax shifted and tilted posterior, the pelvis shifted and tilted anterior, the knees shifted posterior, placing the ankles-feet into plantarflexion relative to the tibiae.

The strategy is to find out what manual cue(s), if applied to a certain location along a particular net of fascial support, result(s) in the most optimal postural change both in quality, quantity, and subjective improvement. However, as opposed to merely attempting to correct posture, which in and of itself has little research to support its value and relevance, it may be more useful to attempt decreasing symptoms or even an awareness of excessive tension (Lemeunier et al. 2018).

If, for example, there is a low level ache in the low back while standing, there is an opportunity to see if a strategic manual cue can reduce or eliminate this discomfort while at the same time improving posture. Because there are many choices where the practitioner may effect manual change, using one or two hands to scan and identify likely regions where the strain distribution may be localized or distributed can expose whole fascial line engagement.

In the example that follows, experience with the aforementioned dysfunctional postural pattern offers the following suggested options:

- Sub-occipital lift: simply adding two fingers to the sub-cranial region by the practitioner as a manual cue for the client to add active lengthening tension to his biotensegrity structure often has immediate global, cascading effects. Among them may be a reduction in magnitude of aberrant patterns in all, most or one fascial plane(s). The reduction in tone or tension in regions under compression are often visually as well as palpably apparent. Concomitantly, you may observe an increase of normalizing stiffness in regions that were slack and

appearing weak or ineffective ("locked long") in maintaining stability (for example, abdominals in the SFN). Often a reduction, if not a complete elimination of pain, ache or stiffness may be reported if the lift is maintained for at least a minute so the client's tissues and fluids have time to adapt to the new positions. Please note that this category of client often has extrinsic eye muscle imbalances that contribute, oftentimes in a major way, to the postural imbalances noted. Redirecting the focus and gaze of the eyes to align with the horizon or more may be needed to complete the re-education, if results are to be long term. However, this subject of assessment and treatment is beyond the scope of this book.

- Clients that respond with major improvements in posture and symptoms with this test will often benefit from an overall global strategy of decompression with FST. In many simple cases like this, the practitioner may stop the assessment and commence table-based FST assessment (described below) and treatment. Experience shows excellent outcomes with this category of client. However, if there are more signs of functional problems in multiple regions and/ or more pain, further assessment is needed before treatment starts.

- Other clients may feel that it is too much effort for them to maintain the postural correction themselves, which may mean other yet unidentified regions are still under compression, thus offering a measure of resistance to the globally intended sub-occipital lift. For instance, the thoracolumbar region may be where it is resisting, which is discussed next. Or, the client may be deconditioned and thus needs endurance training for the fascial nets that hold the body up against the forces of gravity and whatever is required for daily functional activities of living.

- Thoracolumbar shift-lift: when using hands to scan and then identify this region, you will often feel an immediate lack of resilience and response to manual cuing. It feels immobile and locked down, yet with the proper manual lift and shift opposite to the pattern (i.e. superior-anterior) with cued breathing, this mini-treatment often produces an immediate reduction in stiffness locally as well as in pain distally in the lower lumbar spine and/or sacroiliac joint(s). Note also how the bipolar ends at the head-neck and knees respond in this pattern. If there is a better global response to this cue than there was at the sub-occipitals, then this is the more likely region for treatment focus, even though the other areas may still be addressed.

- Knee shift: after testing global responses to manual corrections at the sub-occiput and thoracolumbar regions, those results are compared to manually shifting the knees anteriorly just enough to "soften" them out of a locked knee or hyperextension position that is often actively held. Locking or holding the knees is usually a secondary consequence of what is "not right" above and below those joints, so most clients often require motor re-patterning to work with the rest of the body. The trickle down effect of shifting the knees a little forward will usually correct the excessive plantarflexion in the foot-ankle region unless a significant local restriction is present.

- All of the above: naturally, the client may manifest any combination of the previously described posture faults – or even all of them. The point is to find what may be the

dominant player, do a mini-treatment test to confirm, and proceed from there.

> **NOTE**
>
> 1. Ensure that the client looks straight ahead during all postural assessments and re-education. While this will reduce the tendency for the eyes to have a negative effect on posture, it should be noted that clients should be tested for oculomotor imbalances and/or vestibular disorders if they respond poorly to this assessment.
>
> 2. Posture in sitting should be assessed for all clients that function in that position. This may involve experimenting with a variety of seat heights and other extrinsic ergonomic factors that play a large factor in how the body shapes itself to the work and work environment. This extensive topic is not discussed here.

3. **Local**: when the client does not display a global subjective/objective positive response to static posture testing, a local issue affecting fascial net tension is suspected. Pain or another symptom that does not change is another sign to assess locally. A unilateral fascial net may be insufficiently supportive and be collapsed and be especially dependent on a local, more or less rigid (versus flexible) fixation. For example, this is often seen when only one foot has a pronation dysfunction. You may try to get a global response by using the techniques previously described but usually to no avail, as the pronated foot does not respond.

If verbal or manual cues are used to see if the client can actively supinate the foot but the foot pronates again when it is relaxed, the client has a "flexible fixation." It is flexible in the sense that it can adapt and achieve a new position actively but it is still a fixation, as it returns to an imbalanced, dysfunctional position of function relative to the rest of the body. On the other hand, if the client cannot respond to any cues and the foot remains pronated then they have a "rigid fixation." That does not necessarily mean they need orthotics, only that there is a need for specific manual therapy and motor pattern re-training to get the foot, ankle, and rest of the body to respond to triplanar motion and be capable of successfully adapting to varied movement and terrain challenges.

Continuing this example, it is easy to imagine unilateral pronation or, as practitioners of Structural Integration put it, a medial tilt of the rear and mid-foot with a shift of the lower Deep Front Net (DFN) inferiorly. Imagine using SITTT assessment, verbal cues, and specific touch to manually lengthen the lateral band of the outside arch, but also adding cues to activate and shorten the medial band at the same time, which often helps fascial line engagement even more. As a bonus, the entire DFN responds with facilitation and engagement, lifting the arches of the foot to align and balance the bodyweight in a more neutral position. Often accompanying, related corrections all the way upstream in all nets simultaneously occur. This imagined scenario taken from actual common clinical experience informs the practitioner to focus on those areas of the foot during the FST treatment and re-education part of the session. While clients rarely have just one problem, the treatment will be biased toward the unilateral foot and ankle in manual work and then motorically integrated with the rest of the body during the re-training.

B. Dynamic

Once the fascial nets have been assessed statically, it is time to observe them in movement. As in the static exam above, global before local movements will be assessed. However, the local assessment will seek to differentiate myofascia from joint from nerve issues within fascial nets so that the global context of a problem is always considered.

As researchers and clinicians Shumway-Cook and Woollacott state in their text on motor control: "there is no one theory of motor control that everyone accepts" (2016). Consequently, here movement analysis will be restricted to assessing the quality and quantity of fascial net engagement (as well as the lack of it). Until such time as motor control theories concur and have standard guidelines of practice for all clinicians, the empirical system we discuss here has served and will serve practitioners and their clients very well for quite a long time.

At first, movement may be tested within the standing base of support position and then the challenge increased by moving outside the base of support. That way, added challenges to balance might be minimized and restricted to other specific balance tests. Tensegrity strain is also minimized such that symptoms of pain and/or instability are less likely to be triggered and movement can be better controlled by both client and practitioner to assess pain. Here are two examples of dynamic assessments:

1. Standing full body movements

A. Inside the base of support

- Test full body rotation active movement. This is an excellent functional test primarily of the Spiral Nets beginning in neutral standing, which is the starting position for gait and many other activities of daily living. It also allows you to observe the difference in quality, quantity, and sequencing order of myofascial chain activation skeletal movements, and to see whether any of these has an impact on symptoms such as nerve compression. Easy access and ability to manually test global and local regions facilitate an efficient assessment for the practitioner. Other reasons for using this test include the following:

- o All joints start in neutral posture position, thereby minimizing symptoms from uneven joint loading.
- o Neuromyofasciae start with minimal postural tone and tension activation to minimize symptoms from these regions.
- o End position of active rotation only adds a relatively small amount of tension, compression, and shear across multiple axial body structures for a quick, full body test.
- o SITTT can easily be used to assess/assist/resist local motion or global movement.
- o Provides a good base test from which one may build a matrix of progressive challenge and provocation tests to assist diagnosis.

- When observing movement sequencing, note the relative acceleration/deceleration of the whole body first, then specific regions. Hypomobile joints and/or restricted myofasciae will decelerate much more rapidly in comparison to adequate motion. Hypermobile joints with their excessively lengthened ligaments and attaching myofasciae will naturally go through a greater ROM before decelerating. Strategic assisted manual control – facilitation or inhibition – may be used with SITTT to diagnose problems with motor control and/or whole or regional myofascial lines, joint(s) and nerve(s). Correlative work with these issues using FST on the table will be described later to logically tie assessment and treatment together.

- Whenever possible, initiate the same overall movement from different ends and parts of the body. We all require this movement ability in our lives whether it is used daily or rarely. The following describes the process of initiating movement first from the head and eyes, with respect to what motions should simultaneously occur on the opposite side of that same region:

- o head and eye motion
- o sequential spinal regional and segmental motion, from neck to lumbar
- o innominate anterior and posterior rotation
- o sacral torsion
- o femoral external and internal rotation
- o tibia-fibula external rotation and internal rotation
- o feet supination and pronation.

The same test should be assessed in reverse sequencing, i.e. starting with feet supination and pronation motion. As many relevant movements as possible that can be tested in this manner will make the assessment more comprehensive and inclusive to reveal the most elusive signs and symptoms one is attempting to reproduce. Naturally, other fascial lines may be similarly tested as indicated.

If assessing in a classical ROM-like manner, such as many practitioners do, whole fascia nets of stability and mobility contributing to the efficiency of any motion should always be considered, even if one joint is being tested. In dominant planes of motion, the agonistic net of myofasciae will be observed along with the response of its antagonists and synergists. Finally, with any movement assessment, consideration must be given as to whether the client shows observable stress, indicating that they are trying to deal with a perceived threat. Studies show that the brain is wired for survival and any threat creates a cascade of undesired responses that would be best to avoid during therapy and re-education for most clients.

B. Outside the base of support

If the client does not have a condition (for example, oculomotor, vestibular, etc.) that manifests as a balance disorder, then you may safely test movements outside the base of support. This includes all movements that move the body beyond where the feet are placed. Many positions of function are outside a simple standing or sitting base and may include transitional movements. A common example of a transitional movement that many clients with back and knee pain have trouble with is going from standing to sitting in a car, and vice versa. Movements like this and many others need to be assessed exactly as the client performs them, with the practitioner using the same methods described above using the SITTT method so that it becomes clear what to focus on during the table treatment and follow-up movement re-education.

An easier movement to assess is the squat performed in the sagittal plane. Trainers tend to test squats meant for weightlifting (i.e. keep lumbar spine and pelvis neutral) while others test squats as indigenous people perform them (allowing the lumbar spine to flex and the pelvis to posteriorly rotate). More comprehensive assessments will evaluate both functions.

Squat assessment example:

As a test, it is often helpful to place a circular weight plate, shim or similar object beneath the client's heels to raise them. This simulates added length and confirms whether a shortened or tight Achilles and/or soleus muscle is present, causing an aberrant squat pattern. Trainers and practitioners familiar with this test will confirm that gross aberrant faults – for example, an excessively forward trunk lean – are often immediately corrected. The common solution then is to stretch the soleus/Achilles.

However, it is not specific enough to be the only assessment, as it does not indicate whether the problem is due to:

- gross postural shift anteriorly with excessive weight on forefoot/toes
- posterior ankle joint capsule hypomobility
- subtalar joint hypomobility
- talus posterior glide insufficiency

- plantar fascia shortening
- soleus shortening
- heel pad slide hypomobility
- specific scar tissue restriction in any of the above regions or elsewhere
- over-activation of: toe flexors, plantar intrinsics, soleus, gastrocsoleus, hamstrings, the whole back net of fascia, etc.

It is much more useful for the practitioner to use their hands in particular ways on specific tissues along specific nets of fascia to both test their hypothesis of where and when they think the problem in movement is and how it manifests. This must be done whenever possible in the functional or other position that slightly reproduces symptoms or problems without creating additional, lasting pain or inflammation. When the assessment is conducted in this manner, it is often a rapid process that leads the practitioner to adjust the tensional net of the individual to test whether it results in any improvement in symptoms and/or movement. It also helps the client assess what they may be doing or not doing that is contributing to the problem.

In the squat example, if the practitioner manually differentiates in a test that, for example, assists the posteromedial plantar fascia to lengthen and improves the squat more than everting the calcaneus or posteromedially gliding the talus, then the practitioner empirically knows what to do and where to start. For example, the practitioner may make a clinical decision to get the client on the table to perform specific manual therapy techniques for lengthening the plantar fascia, then return the client to perform the same exact test movement to determine if symptoms and signs improve or not. Barring having precise parameters of evidence-based research available that is pertinent to this case, we have found the previous to be the fastest, most accurate clinical approach for best outcomes in most cases that are commonly classified as orthopedic and musculoskeletal diagnoses, as well as a fair share of neurological cases.

2. Standing (or sitting) extremity movements

Following the logic and sequence of assessment initially described in this chapter – that is Scan-Identify-Test-Treat-Test on Posture-Myofascia-Joint-Nerve (SITTT on PMJN) – it will be assumed for the purposes of this section that posture has already been assessed. Maybe it was the case that the shoulder improved 50% when posture was corrected but the client still has shoulder pain. Then again, maybe posture had nothing to do with it. In either case, you must narrow the focus and assess the shoulder. The order of checking is myofascial nets or connections before joints or nerves.

The fact that the normal daily forces of tensegrity and function have rendered many joint manipulation treatments as temporary and ultimately ineffective lends support to starting assessment and treatment with myofascia. That does not mean, of course, that there aren't times when a direct joint manipulation or some other isolated treatment is definitely indicated as the treatment of choice.

Getting back to the shoulder pain example, manual scanning by experienced practitioners will take them to regions that correlate with familiar patterns they have seen in history taking and assessments of posture and function. Evaluating regions like the pectoralis minor and coracobrachialis (which sit in the chain called the Deep Front Arm Net) is standard for clients with locked short Superficial Front Nets who sit at desks all day. However, if a client, for example, fell on an outstretched hand and has had years of post-traumatic chronic pain in the proximal shoulder along with specific weakness and instability, the assessment takes on an even more characteristic direction. This is certainly true when first scanning myofascia for regions of dysfunction that respond to SSS (Stretching-Shortening-or-Stabilization).

Myofascial testing

With a client history of falling on an outstretched hand, you may try to imagine how an equal and

opposite force from the ground was attenuated by the client. The fact that there is no fracture in our example shows that it was at least absorbed without a strong enough force to break bone. Here, with suggested rationale, are some suggested places to scan-treat-test:

- *Scalene – 1st rib attachment*: shoulder was likely forcibly compressed into adduction-elevation with a large portion of the bodyweight on it. Post-trauma daily positioning to lessen pain may have also contributed to this position. After starting with the central axis of the spine and clearing the neck as a source for problems, the next strategy may be attempting to test lengthening the scalene attachment to the 1st rib. Simultaneously re-testing function and/or pure ROM will quickly determine if this is the best way to begin treatment or not.
- *Levator scapula*: often implicated with other synergists in pathologically elevating shoulder dysfunctions; attempting to lengthen will determine if that helps or not.
- *Coracoclavicular ligaments*: may have been partially or fully disrupted. Shortening the ligaments and assessing the acromioclavicular and other ligaments in the chain will help determine if this is or is not the case. After thoroughly scanning through as many fascial nets as makes sense, you may then test joint connections within or intersecting the lines.

Joint testing

Continuing with the same client example as above, one may imagine severe joint compression from wrist to shoulder that was sustained during the client's fall. Testing decompression or joint capsule traction-lengthening as well as stabilization in a specific plane of movement may be indicated. This was the case with a student in one of our workshops (Frederick & Frederick 2019). When the sternoclavicular joint was stabilized with posterior-inferior compression during active abduction, instability and pain were eliminated as strength and ROM increased.

While lax ligaments and unstable joints may need prolotherapy or surgery as a long-term solution, compressed joints respond quite favorably to decompression or traction during an FST session. Often, increased duration and frequency of repetition are indicated in these kinds of cases and are discussed below in the table assessment section.

In any event, testing joint capsules with stretching, shortening, or stabilization quickly informs the practitioner about which direction the treatment should take.

Nerve testing

This topic is beyond the scope of this book but necessary to mention; we refer you to other authorities on this subject (Shacklock 2005).

Nevertheless, it will be mentioned that as part of the diagnostic process for the most comprehensive assessment and treatment approach, central and peripheral nervous system testing for mobility – slide, glide, tension, compression – must be included. Due to the high degree of manual sensitivity and other skills required, coupled with the high potential to adversely reproduce symptoms, these tests are performed at the end of the assessment. Elusive, non-responsive neurological and mechanical problems are often discovered and helped using neuromyofascial techniques focusing on the multilayered tissues of the nervous system. From our experience, these tests fit in perfectly with the SITTT protocol and are fully compatible with the rest of the assessment.

Movement assessment summary

In general, the more movements become functional and less purely a ROM test, the more neuromyofascial lines are engaged. An example of contrasting tests for shoulder motion versus movement would be having a track and field athlete client do the standard shoulder flexion AROM test and then observe them, ideally with their coach, do javelin throw drills in a field. The first motion generally engages a local shortening contraction of the Superficial and Deep Front Arm Nets and a lengthening contraction of the Superficial and Deep Back Arm Nets. In contrast, throwing a javelin also engages full body Spiral, Functional, and Lateral as well as some other nets. In addition to many other things that are activated in a way that ROM testing does not, the visual, vestibular, and other parts of the nervous system are recruited in unique, task-specific ways that also need to be evaluated to rule out and/or rule in additional aspects affecting function (not discussed in this book).

As noted with the javelin athlete, movement assessment often offers a dizzying number of possibilities of what to observe and where to start. Therefore, to deconstruct and then assess individual whole fascial nets, starting with static posture and progressing to dynamic movements will help simplify the process and organize the flow of the assessment. With experience, one will quickly and accurately begin to understand the integration and intersection of fascial chain dynamics.

Table-based assessment

When imagining FST, the movement of both the client on the table and the practitioner should be considered. If manual therapy were an artistic endeavor, the FST practitioner as artist would be a dancer, moving gracefully and fluidly back and forth, around the table as well as undulating his or her body up and down and side to side. In the ideal scenario, the client is the willing dance partner. The point here is that palpatory literacy in FST is dynamic and must extend, with specific intention and in particular sensorimotor patterns, to and from the communicating neuromyofascial nets of both the practitioner and the client. Surprisingly, the authors have observed that manual therapy professionals find this skill quite a challenge to learn, while trainers and other movement professionals pick up those skills more readily. Despite their comparable lack of static palpatory literacy, movement professionals have the advantage over the practitioners in this particular instance while learning FST movement patterns. Some practitioners find it somewhat of a challenge and unfamiliar to feel while simultaneously moving their body dynamically during FST. Yet becoming skilled at this way of working is required in order to master the FST system. The practitioner's body is, after all, a functional extension of their hands and actually amplifies manual therapy communication, ability, and dexterity. Further, if the practitioner is uncoordinated or lacking in their ability to move in the way that is required in FST, they must go through more practice drills to ensure they master the choreography of FST before treating clients. Those who feel awkward on the dance floor have nothing to fear! FST will soon become an enjoyable part of your manual therapy. This is discussed in more depth in in the next chapters of Section 2.

> **NOTE**
> Table-based movements and specific motions (discussed next), are a progression and may include all or some of passive, active, active-assisted, and resistive patterns.

Passive movement

Traction-oscillation-circumduction (TOC) is the foundational pattern of passive joint and neuromyofascial movement that the practitioner will use to get an initial impression of the client's:

- willingness to release voluntary control
- trust in the practitioner
- neuromyofascial mobility
- neuromyofascial response to movement intended to change:
  - autonomic state of the body, for example, stimulate parasympathetic versus sympathetic nervous system

  - regional tone and tension
  - fascial strain distribution
  - pain
- joint condition and tolerance to movement.

After assessing the client's initial responses to the above, the practitioner will have a therapeutic movement vocabulary for the rest of the session to modulate pain, change tone and tension, and maintain trust and a rapport with the client for more successful outcomes. However, it must be emphasized here that the information gained in this initial assessment is used to create an individualized strategy to the session, which is commonly lacking in traditional assisted stretching.

TOC assessment

Traction

Traction may be used to assess the following (as compared to the contralateral side and referenced against the practitioner's experience with this specific technique):

- whether the joint is hyper- or hypomobile
- whether the neuromyofascia is excessively lengthened, shortened, or immobile
- whether the tissue is or was injured, particularly strains, sprains or other traction events along a particular trajectory
- whether the client's tissue(s) is locally or globally compressed, indicating traction in all of its variations as a key element for treatment.

Oscillation

Used as another means to assess neurological response to movement. This response informs the practitioner about the condition of the tissue:

- whether it is healthy and will tolerate more movement, oscillation, or otherwise
- whether the tissue can "calm down" quickly (in seconds) when oscillation is

used for local pain, global autonomic, or regional tone modulation

- whether the tissue is "fragile" or "irritable" and pain takes minutes or longer to resolve – if at all.

Circumduction

Whenever possible, triplanar movements or circumduction is used, starting with smaller circular movements and, where possible, progressing to larger ones. Assessing both clockwise and counter-clockwise movements will reveal preferential directionality to help refine the evaluation.

The following information is gained from testing circumduction:

- feeling the general mobility of the joint surfaces, capsule and ligaments and determining whether it is satisfactory, needs more stability (hypermobile) or more mobility (hypomobile)
- feeling specific mobility of the joint capsule to determine what particular "corners" or angles of movement need to be stretched and/or compressed in a particular manner, or not
- response to joint mechanoreceptor stimulation
- determine if there is joint or neuromyofascial resistance to passive movement (more details immediately below).

TOC is first performed in the barrier-free, "loose-pack" position of joints and soft tissue. By slowly enlarging the diameter of the circular motions, one will start to encounter resistance to movement, which, as another assessment progression, is described next. (Instructions on how to perform TOC with clients will be discussed in Chapter 5.)

Resistance to passive movement (R1–R3)

Also referred to as "dynamic tissue tension" above, resistance to movement in FST uses a designation

that is familiar to many manual therapy practitioners. The late eminent physiotherapist Geoffrey Maitland extensively described and categorized the phenomena of resistance to passive movement, as evaluated by the manual physiotherapist (Maitland 1986). He developed what he called a movement diagram, as well as a pain diagram to accompany it. Maitland called the first, minor barrier one encounters during passive movement testing of spasm-free resistance R1. The next one is called R2, with this resistance characterized as limiting further movement unless more force is used to push past this barrier. R3 was additionally named and defined by us as the last, often painful, barrier to movement, called the anatomical end range of motion. In this book, the reader is advised and will be instructed never to go past R2 with FST assessments, treatment or exercise prescription.

The concept of R1–R2 can be easily understood by experiencing it on one's own finger. We use this when explaining what makes FST different from other kinds of stretching and jokingly call it the "Frederick Finger of Fascia". Follow along in the accompanying photos.

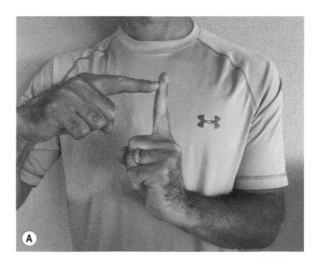

(A)

Figure 4.2a Point one finger up; push with other finger until barrier felt.

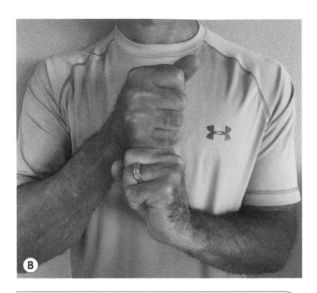

Figure 4.2b **Now grasp finger, pull up to ceiling**

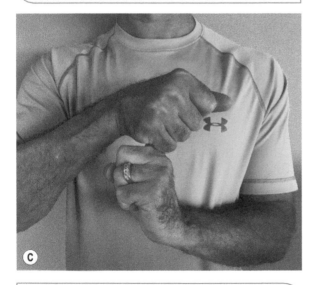

Figure 4.2c **Keep traction as you assist finger extension to next barrier (R2)**

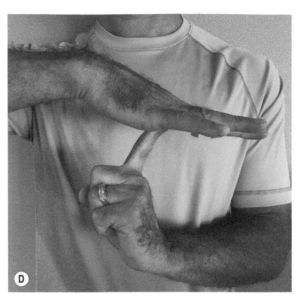

Figure 4.2d **Notice 2–3 times more gain in ROM**

example, tissues that rapidly respond favorably to these movements indicate that FST would be an optimal solution for a particular tissue or fascial net problem, usually within that session. This information will determine how to further individualize the session for best outcomes.

Resisted movement (FST PNF)

As stated in Chapter 2, the Proprioceptive Neuromuscular Facilitation technique of hold or contract-relax, as used in stretching, has a long research history of having the most favorable outcomes for increasing ROM when compared to static and self-stretching. It was also explained that FST uses a modified version of this technique (called FST PNF) to add resistance before an assisted stretch is applied. The following outlines the steps used in the example of a straight leg stretch of the hamstrings:

- Practitioner passively moves client's leg to R2 and instructs client to

TOC is used to assess the quality and quantity of R1–R2 movements and to gain further insight as to whether tissues are responsive or not, hydrated or not, injured or not, and so on. For

inhale and push leg down to table against the practitioner's hand.

- Practitioner allows client to ramp up contraction by permitting up to three degrees of initiating movement.

- After initiating movement, practitioner resists further movement so that further movement becomes an isometric contraction of the hamstrings within the Superficial Back Net of the leg.

- Client stops the isometric contraction and relaxes when he or she needs to exhale.

- Upon exhalation, practitioner passively performs longitudinal traction before stretching into the available range up to the next R2 barrier.

- Classically repeated three times, the number of repetitions is in reality individualized such that when no further gains in range are realized, the stretch at this particular angle is ended and a new angle is chosen.

- The above is repeated at that new angle, if indicated. Information gained during an initial assessment of using FST PNF includes, in general, the quality of neuromyofascial chain engagement/disengagement and, in particular:

  o activation/deactivation quality of targeted myotomes and other muscles within chains

  o determine what tempos (along a spectrum of slow to fast) work best to achieve goals, for example, increasing ROM

  o determine what durations work best

  o determine what frequencies work best

  o determine what intensities work best.

FST PNF is used as an assessment, as treatment and as training. As an assessment, it is used on new clients and at any time a new problem or condition warrants an evaluation to solve a problem. However, as maintenance therapy or training, FST PNF is used primarily to obtain greater increases in end range neuromyofascial chain activation, strength and/or ROM. The next chapters provide a thorough description of the practical FST technique for readers to use with their clients.

Summary

This chapter is essentially about implementing palpatory literacy in a logical sequence of quick and accurate manual assessments in order to guide you to more effective treatments and improved outcomes.

After reviewing the details of using the familiar SOAP format, we broke it down further into a general strategy of assessment of testing tissue by using START (Symptom reproduction-Tissue tenderness-Asymmetry-Range of motion quantity and movement quality-Tissue texture changes). Specificity of accurately and rapidly treating and re-assessing was highlighted in our description of SITTT (Scan-Identify-Treat-Test-Treat again). Detailed practical examples were provided to help guide you in learning the process. The testing part of SITTT was further subdivided into using SSS (Stretch-Shorten-Stabilize), a quick method of testing to see if imposing immediate change to a region of the body net of fascia will affect function positively, in order to quickly direct your treatment.

A discussion of assessment flow followed, directing you to try using SITTT to get positive global before local response to treatment and then move from static tests to dynamic tests of function. We provided a logical ordering for this by using PMJN (Posture-Myofasciae-Joint-Nerve) as the preferred sequence of assessment.

Table-based assessment was then introduced starting first with passive movement testing using TOC (Traction-Oscillation-Circumduction). TOC is the foundational pattern of passive joint and neuromyofascial movement response. We discussed resistance to passive movement, describing how to use the concepts of R1–R3 to help guide you to accurately assess tissue dynamically. Resisted movement using FST modified PNF (FST PNF) was then discussed in detail so as to provide you with a good foundation to understand and practice manual techniques in the following chapters.

Finally, it should be noted that all of the previous assessments are conducted within the biopsychosocial model so that we take into account as many relevant factors as possible that may impact the care, treatment, and outcomes of our clients.

References

Chaitow L (ed.) (2015) Positional Release Techniques, 4th edn. Edinburgh: Churchill Livingstone Elsevier.

Frederick A, Frederick C (2019) Certified Fascial Stretch Therapist Level 1, 2 and 3 workshop manuals.

Gibbons P, Tehan P (2016) Manipulation of the Spine, Thorax and Pelvis, 4th edn. Edinburgh: Elsevier.

Jensenius AR (2011) Difference between the terms movement and motion. [Online] (http://www.arj.no/2011/10/02/difference-between-the-terms-movement-and-motion/).

Lemeunier N, Jeoun EB, Suri M, Tuff T, Shearer H, Mior S, Wong JJ, daSilva-Oolup S, Torres P, D'Silva C, Stern P, Yu H, Millan M, Sutton D, Murnaghan K, Côté P (2018) Reliability and validity of clinical tests to assess posture, pain location, and cervical spine mobility in adults with neck pain and its associated disorders: Part 4. A systematic review from the cervical assessment and diagnosis research evaluation (CADRE) collaboration. Musculoskeletal Science and Practice 38 128–147.

Maitland GD (1986) Vertebral Manipulation, 5th edn. Oxford: Butterworth-Heinemann.

Myers TW (2014) Anatomy Trains: Myofascial meridians for manual and movement therapists, 3rd edn. Edinburgh: Churchill Livingstone Elsevier.

Shacklock M (2005) Clinical Neurodynamics: A New System of Musculoskeletal Treatment. Edinburgh: Elsevier.

Shumway-Cook A, Woollacott MH (2016) Motor Control: Translating research into clinical practice, 5th North American edn. Philadelphia, PA: Wolters Kluwer.

Wade DT, Halligan PW (2017) The biopsychosocial model of illness: A model whose time has come. Clinical Rehabilitation. 31 (8) 995–1004.

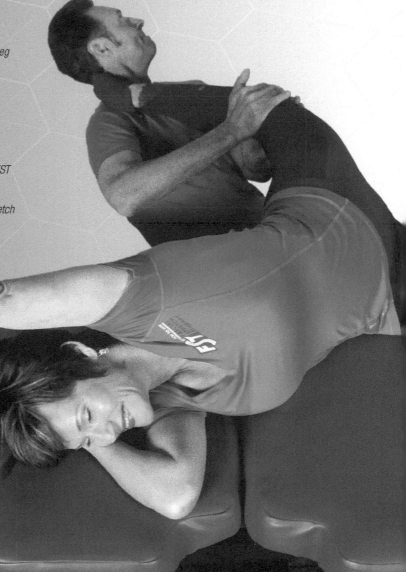

Chapter 5 FST – Lower Body Technique

Key Concepts for Technique

Chapter 6 FST – Upper Body Technique

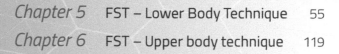

Key Concepts for Technique

Introduction

For experienced practitioners, some of the concepts in this chapter will be familiar. Nonetheless, we felt it crucial and necessary to include them. We share our philosophy, our tips for success, proper body mechanics, and specific instructions on how best to perform our technique. We use our Ten Principles (described in detail in Section 1) to correlate these concepts for better understanding.

The Ten Fundamental Principles of FST

1. Synchronize **breathing** with movement.
2. Tune **nervous system** to current conditions.
3. Follow a logical **order.**
4. Achieve range of motion **gain** *without* **pain**.
5. Stretch **neuromyofascia**, not just muscles.
6. Use **multiple** planes of **movement**.
7. Target the entire **joint**.
8. Get maximal lengthening with **traction**.
9. Facilitate body **reflexes** for optimal results **(PNF)**.
10. Adjust stretching to current **goals**.

All of the principles are applied to the technique and are not done in any specific order. When we teach our hands-on workshop we demonstrate the practical relevance of these guidelines. They are not just theoretical but have an extremely useful application as well. The philosophy and theory of the principles were described in Chapter 3. Here they will be outlined differently for the specific practice of FST technique.

If you truly embrace all of the principles when you perform the technique, you will have excellent results. They have stood the test of time not only for us but also for thousands of our students.

A term we use is the StretchWave™. This is a metaphor used to help people visualize a stretch as being made up of undulations of movement coordinated with proper breathing. It comes from observing that many physiological and kinesiological processes in the body occur in waves, from the light waves that stimulate the retina in vision to the pulsing waves of the blood in arteries and veins. See also undulating stretching.

Practical guide to implementing the Ten Principles

NOTE
You are referred back to Chapter 3 if you need more details on any principle.

---

1. Breathing

Breathing is a crucial component in successful stretching, for both the client and the practitioner. Breathe together and be aware that if the practitioner is not breathing well it often translates to the client not breathing well.

2. Nervous system

We use combination of movement we refer to as TOC in order to "talk" to the tissue. This stands for: traction, oscillation, and circumduction. It uses a combination of breathing cues to either relax (down-regulate) or excite (up-regulate) the client's nervous system. TOC is used in a slow or fast manner, just like the StretchWave™.

Traction

Physically decompress and create space in the joint using your hands or body. Contact with the entire neuromyofascial net through traction lengthens the tissue.

Oscillation

Movement that has a vibratory effect with a rhythmic motion: it can be back and forth, side to side, up and down, in and out, or any combination of these. It can be used to calm down a nervous system, moving the client into the parasympathetic state, or amp up a nervous system, shifting the client into the sympathetic state. Most pain that arises from factors such as unintentionally overstretching or pinching a structure can be relieved in seconds with immediate oscillation.

Circumduction

There are six reasons why we use circumduction in FST:

1. To warm up and thin out synovial fluid in the joint.
2. To assess the feel of the joint and possible impingements.
3. To assess feel of the tissue and check for imbalances.
4. To see if the client is going to give up control and allow us to move them.
5. To increase overall relaxation in joint and entire body.

6. To build trust and rapport with the client. This is very important! Smooth oscillations calm the nervous system. Jiggling, gyrating, yanking movements are jarring to the nervous system. Rapid movement wakes up the nervous system.

3. Order

- Begin at the core of the body to unlock the restrictions first before moving to the extremities.
- Stretch one-joint muscles (bent) before two-joint muscles (straight).
- Start at the deepest innervated structures of the body – the joint – and progressively move all the way through to the distal ends of neuromyofascial chains.

4. Gain without pain

- The risk of causing pain means the possibly losing trust and potential injury. There should be a stretch awareness, but never pain.
- "No pain, no strain!" is one of our fundamental credos. Movement is gained through finesse, not force.
- Less is more – don't overstretch and cause the rebound effect.
- We believe that it is important for the client to understand what a good stretch should feel like and not that it should never hurt.
- You always want client making "aahs" (happy sounds) before they make "oohs" (stretch awareness).

5. Neuromyofascia

Consider the following when practicing FST:

- Think neuromyofascia and shift out of the mindset of engaging with specific muscles.

- When stretching, think global not local. Consider entire continuities of neuromyofascial lines and all the tissue contained within, not just isolated regions.
- Look at the body from a three dimensional perspective – from the inside out. Think: micro macro and macro micro.
- The irrefutable fact that is that it is impossible to separate one tissue from another – it is all intertwined and interdependent.
- Think of adding layers as you stretch into and across tissue: joint capsule, one joint, multiple joints, fascial, neural all the way to two or more practitioners stretching a client along multiple planes, in opposite directions.

6. Multiple planes of movement

- Explore all possible movements – remember it is a dance!
- Play with angles to find all of the tight fibers.
- Change the angle or level to find different fibers and tissue restrictions.
- Move in 3–5 degree increments around the body, like the sweep hand on a watch.

7. Joint

- Proprioceptively, the knee specifically needs contact – hand and/or body placement around the knee – for a sense of security. This makes the joint feel safe and stable, rather than hanging unsupported in space.
- Gently cradle the knee instead of grabbing or gripping it.
- In side lying moves, make sure you are supporting the client's knee and ankle (keep in line with knee-femur and tibia). Dropping the ankle below the knee can cause tweaking in the knees.
- If the joint has been stretched open for a while, then close it; or if it has been closed for a while, open it. Joints don't like to be in one position for too long.

8. Traction

TIP

"When in doubt, traction it out!"
Traction is the cornerstone of FST. Consider the following features and benefits:

1. Opens the joint capsule and space, decompresses the joint.
2. Creates conditions for optimal mobility of all joint structures.
3. Releases adhesions in joint capsule and other connective tissues.
4. Achieves neuro-reflexive release of the joint capsule being tractioned, as well as neighboring structures – some of which may also cross that joint.
5. Increases endorphin release.
6. Reduces pain.
7. Allows maximal lengthening of all the connective tissues.
8. Eliminates joint compression (jamming or pinching) while stretching.
9. Targets fascial components deep inside joint capsule, ligaments, tendons, muscles, and neural tissues.
10. Dramatically improves the effectiveness of ROM increases and flexibility gains.

Traction points

- Use traction in all positions to find ROM.
- Use your body to traction and very rarely your arms.
- Use it to transition and move from one position to the next.

- Slow down, make sure your angle/position is correct for both you and your client.
- Traction can be done at varying degrees and angles – through multiple planes.
- Hand placement during traction (i.e. under versus over) is important, especially during the straight leg segment.
- When tractioning through any joint, make sure to target only the intended joint and be cautious of hypermobile joints.
- We like to say "When in doubt, traction it out!". This means use traction when:
  o the client feels joint or tissue pinch
  o you forget what to do next
  o the client cannot relax
  o the client gets a spasm, etc.

Don't use traction on acute injuries or in conditions of hypermobility or laxity.

9. PNF

Described in detail earlier, it is the flowing dance of two people and their respective neuromyofascial systems moving in therapeutic harmony. Each dance is unique to the practitioner and the client. Uses specific simple cues (verbal, tactical, importance of hand placement). It is key not to touch the opposite side of the body or you send a neurological signal to the wrong area.

10. Current goals

- Know what the current goal is and keep treatments on track with it.
- Change the goals in order to continue moving ahead to successfully achieve them.
- Adapt sequencing to your client and what their tissue needs are at a particular moment, not to what is on your agenda.

- Apply asymmetrical dosing of stretching, for example, 2:1 (or, if needed, 3 or 4:1) ratio to correct side-to-side ROM imbalances, where ROM unilaterally is remarkably decreased.

Range of motion evaluation

Explanation of resistance of the tissue feel

The purpose is to get a passive sense of soft tissue resistance to movement and to identify the type of tissue (joint capsule, ligament, neuromyofascial unit or chain) that is responsible for movement restrictions or other aberrations. The purpose of the ROM assessment is to get a sense of when soft tissue starts to resist the passive movement being directed by the practitioner. The first response of passive resistance to PROM is called Resistance 1 or simply, R1. This occurs when the practitioner feels or senses the first barrier encountered, as one takes up increasingly more PROM. R1 can occur at the relative start of the ROM or may occur toward the expected end or anywhere along that spectrum. The feel of R1 can be soft or hard or somewhere in between. It can have a gooey, almost nondescript feel, as in some long practicing yoga practitioners who have reduced the gamma gain of the muscle as well as over-lengthened their connective tissue by excessive stretching. R1 in this body type will occur toward the expected end of the ROM and, in some, it will actually coincide with the anatomical limit of joint motion. On the other side of the spectrum, R1 can have a wiry, guitar string feel, such that it springs into your hand almost suddenly, which usually occurs at the relative beginning of the ROM. We generally see this in the following client types: highly strung, massively stressful life, cannot give up being the one in control, highly nervous and or anxious, distrustful. Many disorders of the nervous system or some diseases of the connective tissue system may also have these or similar characteristics, but those topics are beyond the scope of this book.

R2 or Resistance 2, is the second response to the PROM evaluation. After you note where R1 occurs, proceed to increase the ROM until you feel the tissue suddenly start to slow down the movement. Any further movement after this point will elicit maximal resistance (R3) from the tissue (and probably a look of pain or high alert from the client) and possibly a reflex reaction that contracts the muscle to prevent further lengthening of the tissue. Naturally, this scenario is undesirable and can be avoided if the practitioner is attentive to the feel of tissue under tension, as well as to the reaction and response of the client.

Resistance to Traction (RT) occurs during the actual stretching phase of the session, not during the evaluation or ROM phase. RT can conceptually be thought of as "enhanced R2," meaning that the second barrier felt during PROM is explored with the addition of two simultaneously occurring components, traction and increased ROM. For example, when working to increase bent knee hip flexion at R2, we first micro-traction, then add more flexion while maintaining the traction.

- Move into starting position for ROM without being in a rush to get into the stretch.
- The ROM check needs to be just that, a check – no stretching yet.
- It needs to be the client's end ROM, not what is shown in the book.
- Know where R1 is for your client and stay there during the evaluation and warm-up. Check in with your client if you are not certain.

Breathing technique

The importance of using the breath to maximize gains in the tissue and also to help control the desired nervous system is the second of the Ten Principles. This can be easily achieved by the practitioner and client breathing together to achieve synchronized movement and flow. The basic rule with FST is to exhale into all movements, be it finding the ROM or into the stretch post PNF contraction. An inhalation is taken for both the brief concentric and then isometric contraction component during PNF.

The following is a detailed explanation of how FST PNF is performed for the first move in the routine. We use part of the Superficial Back Net as one example, which targets the gluteus maximus and proximal attachment hamstrings. It represents how it is executed through the entire technique.

PNF technique

This technique uses a modified form of PNF we call FST PNF to help differentiate it from traditional and other forms of PNF. In FST PNF, the client contracts targeted muscles with as little as 5% of their strength and up to 20% (versus traditionally 50–100%) and holds the contraction for approximately three to four seconds (versus six to ten seconds), for a more effective relaxation response. We use comfortable straps to stabilize the limb that is not being worked on, thus facilitating complete relaxation of the person being stretched and enhancing the effectiveness of the actions of the practitioner.

Other key differences are that traction is used to assess the ROM in the tissue before the stretching begins. It is also gently used throughout the stretching. Pain is never allowed and is considered a negative response. The practitioner and client move together as if in a dance, with perpetual undulating movements through the session. For a list of 18 reasons that make FST PNF different, please see Principle 9 in Chapter 3.

FST PNF sample sequence

1. Begin with the client's leg placed comfortably on your body, draped over your shoulder and with the weight of their leg resting on your back. Their other leg is normally secured by stabilization straps for this routine.

TIP

> If you don't have straps, you will have to modify accordingly: use your other hand to stabilize when possible, use an assistant, or have the client perform active stabilization.

2. Make sure your own body mechanics are good (you are also relaxed and in a comfortable position).

3. The client and practitioner both inhale together. You will breathe together for the entire session.

4. Using your body (not just your hands) to lift their leg, traction their femur up out of the socket and then take their leg into their barrier of resistance (R1, described previously). Their knee remains bent, as the focus in this case is proximal tissue.

5. The practitioner gives a gentle hand tap to the back of their hamstring for the PNF cue. Ask them to inhale and press back and meet your resistance. The client performs a slow and gradual concentric contraction of the hamstrings and gluteus maximus for just a few degrees of movement into hip extension and with as little as 5–20% of their strength for the duration of the inhalation.

The reason there is such a large variance in the percentage of the contraction is because it depends on the strength of the client as well as the practitioner. The area of the body being targeted also influences it; for example, the neck will use a lighter contraction than the leg. Finally, there is a spectrum of contraction intensities that the practitioner will need to experiment with in order to find the best response to whatever the intent is – increase ROM, reduce tone, etc. This "experiment time" is greatly reduced with practice and experience.

6. After the concentric contraction is performed for a few degrees, the client continues the same inhalation while being cued to hold an isometric contraction, as they firmly meet the resistance provided by the practitioner for about two more seconds. The contraction is then ramped down smoothly until the targeted region completely relaxes.

7. On the exhalation, the practitioner increases the traction of the femur upward out of the hip joint and creates space between the pelvis and the femur, maintaining the traction while increasing the stretch to the next tissue barrier, called R2.

8. This is where the concept of the StretchWave™ is used – like the rise and fall of a wave. The traction up is the rise and movement forward into flexion is the fall.

9. Increased ROM in hip flexion is gained by hooking and carrying the femur upward with your body and hands, thereby enabling deeper and further hip flexion motion. This should look like the StretchWave™ (described in Chapter 3). The traction should be applied at the peak of the wave movement. Flowing into the new –found ROM is likened to the sea washing over the shore after the wave builds into a peak. Use words like "up, out, and down" when you move in unison with your client.

10. Repeat PNF two or more times as indicated by client response, moving a few degrees out into abduction with each PNF pass to a new angle and targeting different, adjacent fibers of tissue.

Repeat the series until you have moved through all the possible angles and fibers to get an optimal fascial stretch of the tissues. Remember: never cause pain or push past appropriate levels of indicated stretch movements. Less is more and patience is important. Always listen to the client's tissue!

The treatment table routines in Chapters 5 and 6 are presented the way we progress through an actual session with a client. They can be done in entirety or in smaller segments for emphasis. What makes the patterns unique is the flow and sequence of movements from the core of the body out to the extremities.

There are also several signature moves such as the "Sack of Buns" and the "Glute Swoop." While developing the technique in the world of athletics, I discovered that it was all about unlocking the tightness around and in the hips. This is why I focused so intently on the four key muscle groups of the lower body. This group consists of the gluteal complex including the six deep rotators, iliopsoas complex, quadratus lumborum, and latisimus dorsi.

Tips for the practitioner's success

The two most important tips are:

1. Listen to your intuition and never, ever go against your gut feelings!
2. Our brain is wired for survival first and foremost, so it is imperative the client always feels safe and that the practitioner is never perceived as a threat. Trust takes time to develop and can be broken in an instant.

More tips

- Less is more. You can always increase the stretch but it is difficult to undo overstretching.

- It takes time and patience to learn to listen and understand the tissue. Go easy on yourself and your skill level. It has taken 30 years to develop this technique and we are still learning every single day from each and every client and student!
- Patience and practice ... slow down and keep listening.
- Listen with your heart, not just your brain to tune into your clients' bodies.
- Don't let your eyes do all your seeing; close them and see what happens.
- When you are in the right position, the stretch movement comes naturally and just flows. If not, it feels awkward to you and to the client!
- Remember to visualize the StretchWave™ throughout the session. Think of moving heel to toe (like tai chi movement) as you move through the stretch wave.
- If you feel like you're working too hard, you are.
- It takes energy, patience and skill to pay attention – not just physical force.
- Own the technique. Play with it. Keep it within the general context and make it yours.
- Remember, we are just bringing our client's bodies back into balance.

Communication

- Work *with* your client not against them. Practitioner intent is a crucial component. Know the power is in listening and working together as a team.
- Be clear in your intention.
- Be clear about the client's goals or concerns for each session. Check in with your client.
- Pay attention to client's verbal cues, facial expressions, and body language.
- Let the client's tissue tell you what it needs. It will talk to you; your job is to listen.

- Don't let the client convince you to deepen a stretch because they think they can go farther when your sense is that the stretch is already at the correct intensity for the best results.
- Be clear and simple in your cueing of PNF.
- Ask for feedback from client. Give communication cues to get specific information:
  - Where do you feel that stretch?
  - On a scale of 1–10?
  - Any pinching?
- Use different ways to elicit feedback (because people don't necessarily know what they're supposed to feel like or be experiencing).
- There is a difference in brain wave patterns between talking and silence. Encourage clients to be where they need to be to accept what you're doing. If their eyes are closed, don't talk; listen to what their bodies are telling you. Let them find their happy place.

Body mechanics

- The golden rule is: if the practitioner feels comfortable and relaxed in their position and the client is relaxed and not in pain – everything works.
- Make the technique your own and don't worry about getting into the perfect position as this will change depending on the size and flexibility of each client as well as the practitioner.

Personal adaptations

- There are no exact hand or leg placements for the practitioner. Position yourself for your ease and comfort. Find what works for you. If you are uncomfortable or in pain, the client senses it and is unable to relax.

> **NOTE**
> Please note that the majority of the photos in the practical section show a petite practitioner and a tall client. The instructions are also for the biomechanics of petite practitioner and a tall client. Therefore, make necessary adjustments of table height, body mechanics, and client positioning to make it work for you.

Position tips for body, legs, and hands have many possible variations:

- The closer your body is to, and the more contact you have with, the client, the better you will be able to read the tissue.
- Use your whole body (feet, hip action, etc.) – not just your hands. This enhances the client's sense of security and thus their ability to relax.
- Always adapt your own body positions according to each client. Your positioning may change depending on the size and flexibility of your client.
- Positioning: is KEY – small adaptations can make a huge difference.
- Use soft, relaxed hands. Don't grip roughly.
- You are not just moving your client, you are moving with them.
- For better results, and less soreness and fatigue in your own body, use leverage rather than pulling and pushing (strong arming) your client. Always release the stretch through a neutral pathway and a different plane – don't re-contract what you have just lengthened.
- Remember always: finesse not force.

The text in Chapters 5 and 6 is broken down into logical steps for you to follow:

Goal: What is the intent of the specific movement and target tissue?

Client position: What is the position of the client on the table (or couch)?

Practitioner: What is the practitioner's position and what do they do?

ROM: What is the movement needed to find ROM?

Traction: What is the target area and how does the practitioner achieve it?

PNF: What does the client do?

PNF cues: What does the practitioner say to the client to verbally cue contraction?

Stretch: What is the target area? What is the movement needed and what does the practitioner do to increase the stretch or vary other parameters?

For simplicity's sake, we have placed all of the same key components at the beginning of this chapter. They apply to the entire technique of the FST system outlined in the rest of the chapter. So for instance, instead of writing the breathing cues for each stretch, they are stated once from the start. The same is true for PNF sequences.

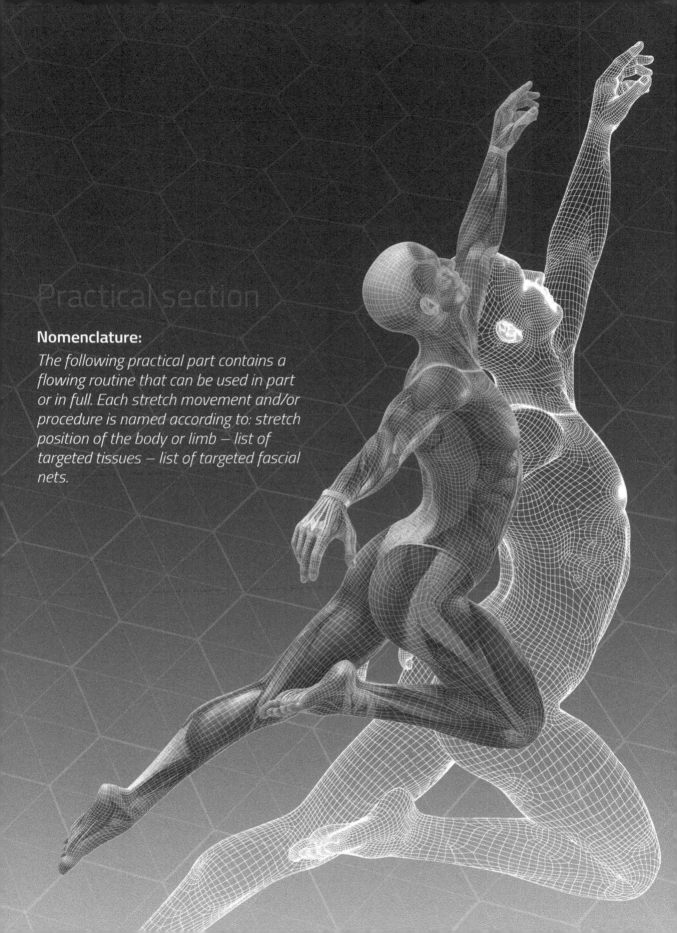

Practical section

Nomenclature:

The following practical part contains a flowing routine that can be used in part or in full. Each stretch movement and/or procedure is named according to: stretch position of the body or limb — list of targeted tissues — list of targeted fascial nets.

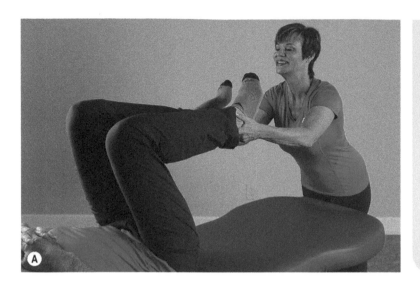

Figure 5.1
Hip clearance

A. General Assessment

1. Major observations

Goal: To look at the client from the overall perspective. To assess the client's body before beginning a session.

Client position: Supine and relaxed on table. Arms are down, alongside the client's body.

Practitioner: Standing at the foot of the table.

2. Hip clearance move

Goal: To ensure the client is aligned correctly on the table. To assess the passive flexion of lumbar spine, pelvis, and hips.

Client position: Supine.

Practitioner:

- Grasp the heels and lift both of the client's legs off the table.
- Bend both knees toward their chest, then straighten out the legs and slowly bring them back down to the table.
- Make sure client remains relaxed and does not help you as you return to the starting position.

- Reason for move: eradicates false positive leg length discrepancies (LLD) due to poor positioning on table.

3. Leg length check

Goal: To check bilateral medial malleoli for LLD.

Client position: Supine with arms down at their sides.

Practitioner:

- Standing at the foot of the table.
- Place your thumbs under medial malleoli edges, resting other fingers on feet.
- Look straight down to check leg length and compare.
- Frequently, the short leg is the dominant leg, especially in athletes.

4. Double leg traction

Goal: To feel for tension and restrictions throughout client's entire fascial net.

Client position: Supine and relaxed with arms at their sides.

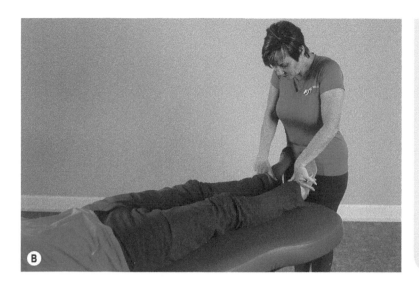

Figure 5.1b
Leg length check

Breath: Both the client and practitioner inhale to prepare for the movement and then exhale into the movement together.

Practitioner:

- Hold both heels in the palms of your hands and gently wrap your fingers around the rest of the feet.
- Lift both of the client's extended legs with traction at 10–20° hip flexion.
- Engage your core and bend your knees slightly.
- Lean back with your body, stay relaxed.
- Where do you feel the client's tension and/or lack of tissue yield/elasticity?

Traction: Through both legs.

5. Single leg traction

Goal: To assess the hip joint capsule by performing moderate traction until slight elastic give is felt in the tissue. To find their specific "sweet spot" which is the optimal open joint position for traction. To decompress joint and create more space.

Client position: Supine and relaxed with arms at their sides.

Practitioner: Standing at the foot of the table.

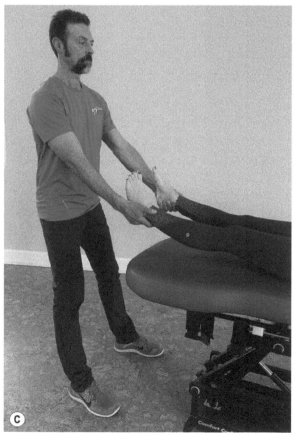

Figure 5.1c
Double leg traction

- Position client's leg approximately 20° flexion and abduction, with a slight external rotation of the femur.
- Hold their heel with the outside hand and wrap your other hand around the inside of their mid-foot moving foot into dorsiflexion. If this hand position does not feel secure to you, or the client's ankle is hypermobile and/or painful, try another variation by wrapping both hands around the malleoli and above the ankle joint (shown in Figures 5.5a and b).

Traction: Relax your own body. Lean back with your body to achieve the traction. Do not pull with your arms; rather, let your body do the work.

Repeat traction three times with a bit more force each time, as indicated.

NOTE
1. Do not pull, yank or try to "pop" the hip. If the hip spontaneously manipulates during traction, do not repeat this specific traction again.
2. Do not try to manipulate the other hip (unless you are licensed to do so); just repeat same on other side as noted above.
3. Hypermobile and/or painful ankle joints require the practitioner to anchor hands above the joint or otherwise stabilize it manually.

Hip capsule end feel:

Normal = ±50% elastic give

Hypomobile = < 50%

Hypermobile = > 50%

Repeat: On the other leg.

Oscillate: Both legs before moving on to the lateral line check for relaxation. Gently move legs in and out of internal and external rotation.

Gently and slightly shake legs up and down.

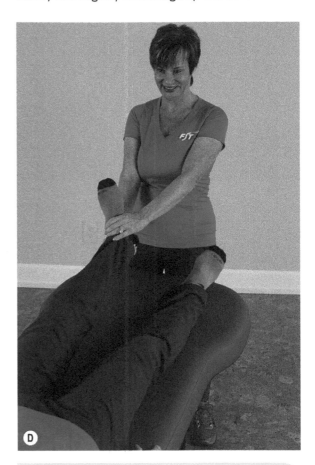

Figure 5.1d
Single leg traction

6. Check lateral movement (moving to the practitioner's left side)

Goal: To assess the client's ROM on the lateral side of their body and to ascertain where they may be restricted as you move them laterally.

Client position: Supine with arms at their side.

Practitioner:

- Lift both of the client's extended legs with traction at 10–20° again.
- Hold both of their heels in the palms of your hands and gently wrap your fingers around their heels.
- Engage your core and bend your knees slightly.
- Move slowly to the left until the client's movement stops.
- If their hip begins to roll up off the table you have reached the end of their ROM.

Traction: Lean back with your body, stay relaxed.

From the last position

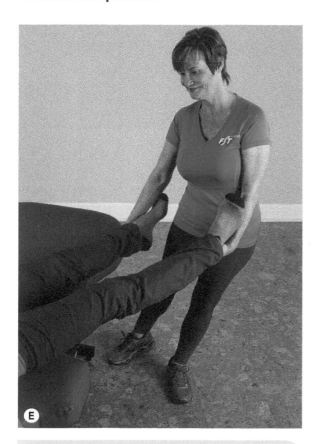

Figure 5.1e
Lateral net check – walking to the right

Goal: To increase ROM in lateral lumbopelvic hip region, especially lateral QL, TFL/IT band and all tissue along lateral net.

Practitioner:

- Place the client's left leg (the bottom one) on your hip or quad as you move to your left.
- Lift their top leg higher, holding at their heel.
- Place your inside hand on their medial malleolus and anchor it to your thigh on your inside leg.
- Increase ROM by increasing lateral flexion of their opposite side.
- Use your body to lean way from the table and not your arms to feel the tissue response and end feel.

Traction: Keep tractioning out as you move.

Think of the traction as if you are moving together in an arc away from the table, then up toward the top of the table.

Repeat: On the other side.

Caution: Return to start position if anything like the following occurs: any sensation of pain or paresthesias which may come from unidentified disc or nerve issues.

ROM check

Before you begin stretching, it is important to have a good benchmark for improvement before treatment commences.

Goal: To assess initial ROM for later re-assessment.

Client position: Supine.

Practitioner:

- Perform a straight leg raise (SLR) PROM to R1.
- Use the heel of your hand to lift the client's leg, keeping your fingers relaxed.
- Use your lats; keep your arm straight to help.

ROM: Make a note of what the ROM is to start off with.

Repeat: On the other leg.

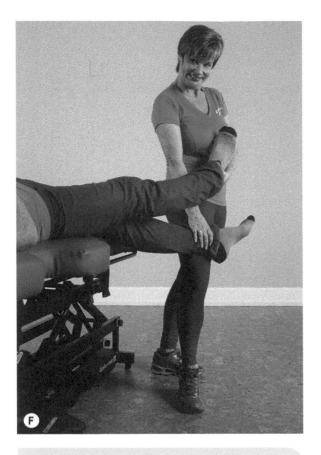

Figure 5.1f
Lateral net with crossed legs

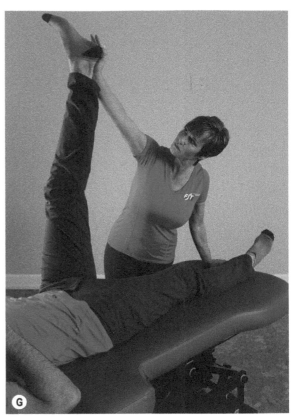

Figure 5.1g
Straight leg raise (ROM check)

The Anatomy Train Nets will be included in each group of movements in an abbreviated manner:

LN	Lateral Net
SN	Spiral Net
FN	Functional Net
DFN	Deep Front Net
SBN	Superficial Back Net
SFN	Superficial Front Net
SFAN	Superficial Front Arm Net
DFAN	Deep Front Arm Net
SBAN	Superficial Back Arm Net
DBAN	Deep Back Arm Net

B. Range of Motion Evaluation Warm-up and FST PNF Stretch – Bent Leg Single Joint

Back net and deep front net (SBN, DFN)

Multiple plane soft tissue ROM evaluation and stretch guidelines:

- Move to **R1 only** for warm-up before moving into stretch.
- **Exhale** into all ROM increases and stretches.
- **Inhale** into all of preparations and PNF contractions.
- Use **gentle traction** throughout ROM and stretches.
- Move in 3–5° increments as you assess tissue for ROM and stretching.

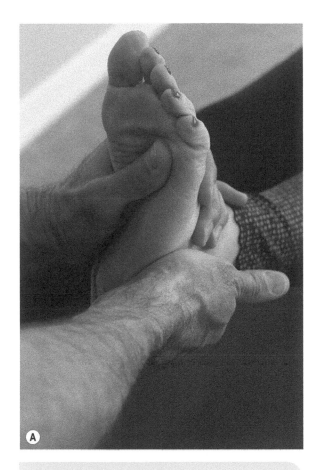

Figure 5.2a
Hand positions for practitioner

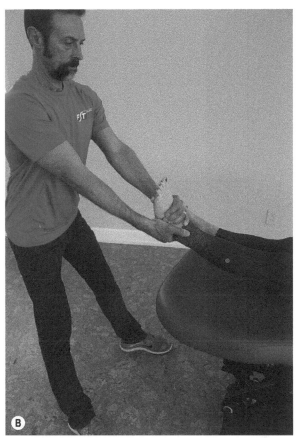

Figure 5.2b
Single leg traction

Goal: To assess the hip joint capsule and perform moderate traction until slight elastic give is felt in the tissue.

To find the client's individual "sweet spot" which is the optimal open joint position for traction.

Client position: Supine and relaxed with arms at their sides.

Practitioner: Standing at the foot of the table.

- Position the client's leg approximately 20° flexion and abduction, with a slight external rotation of the femur.

- Hold their calcaneus with outside hand and wrap your inside hand around the

mid-foot, moving foot into dorsiflexion. If this hand position does not feel secure to you, try another variation (alternatives shown in Figures 5.3a and 5.3b).

- Hold their calcaneus with outside hand and wrap your inside hand over the top of their ankle and hold lateral ankle.

Be careful to not allow their foot to move into plantar flexion with top hand pressing down.

Traction: Relax your body. Lean back using your body weight to achieve the traction. Do not pull with your arms – let your body do the work.

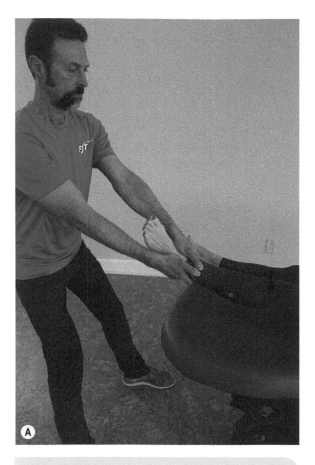

Figure 5.3a
Traction option

1. Circumduction

Goal: See the six reasons to use circumduction in the tip box.

TIP · *We use circumduction in FST to:*

1. Warm up and thin out synovial fluid in the joint.
2. Assess for impingements in the joint.
3. Check for imbalances in the tissues.
4. See if the client is willing to give up control and allow us to move them.
5. Relaxation.
6. And importantly, to build trust and rapport.

Client position: Supine with their left leg bent 90° at the hip and knee, their ankle resting on your shoulder.

The right leg is now under the straps on the table with two straps above the knee and two below.

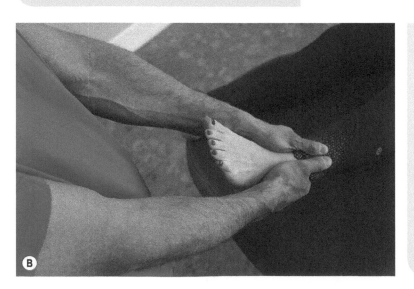

Figure 5.3b
Traction optional hand placement

Use your body by lifting your torso upward and press your foot into the floor for leverage. Remember it's not your hands doing the work but your entire body!

2. Hip/knee flexion – hamstrings, glutei, lumbosacral – SBN, FN

Goal: Target tissues lying within the SBN, FN: proximal hamstrings, glutei, lumbosacral region; also posterior hip joint capsule; hip flexors lying within the DFN in opposite hip in clients with less mobility.

Client position: Supine with their leg relaxed and resting over your shoulder and on your upper back.

Practitioner:

- From the last position, stand up and get into a lunge position with your outside leg forward and your inside leg at the back.
- Lower your torso toward the table to get up under the client's leg.
- Slide your left (inside) shoulder into the back of their knee and wrap the rest of your arm around the leg, securing without squeezing it.
- Be careful not to hit any trigger points with a bony shoulder (you may want to ask the client).

> **NOTE**
> Please note the system of FST was developed around the concept of the client being stabilized with straps for better leverage and control for the practitioner. The straps allow a much deeper stretch and facilitate deeper relaxation in the client. If you don't have straps, you will have to modify accordingly: use your other hand to stabilize when possible, use an assistant, or have the client perform active stabilization.

Practitioner:

- Sit on the same side of the table and place your outside foot firmly on the floor.
- Place your hands on both sides of the client's knee and rest their leg on your shoulder.
- Slide up with your hips and get under their knee with your shoulder.
- Make small slow gentle circles in both directions until you accomplish all six reasons to circumduct noted in the tip box.

Traction: Traction their femur up and out (of hip socket).

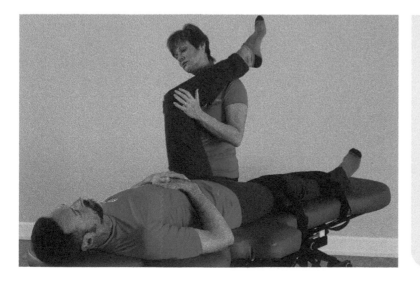

Figure 5.4
Circumduction (up and out)

- Hold onto the side of the table with your right hand.
- Keep your shoulders and torso lowered down.

ROM: changes by increasing hip flexion.

Traction: Traction up (out of socket and toward their head).

Lift their leg up using your legs and torso and not just your arm.

Press off your back foot for power.

To increase the traction press down into the table with your hand as you use your legs to lift their femur up and out.

PNF:

- The client and practitioner both inhale together and breathe together for the entire session.
- The practitioner gives a gentle hand tap to the back of their hamstring for the PNF cue. The client performs a slow and gradual concentric contraction of hamstrings and gluteus maximus with as little 5% and up to about 20% of their strength for about one second. They are allowed to move a few degrees into hip extension. The reason there is such a large variance in the percentage in the contraction is because it depends on the strength of the client as well as the practitioner. It is also influenced by the area of the body being targeted, for example, the neck will use a lighter contraction than the leg.
- Then the contraction changes into an isometric one as it meets the resistance provided by the practitioner for about two more seconds. The contraction then smoothly decreases in its intensity.
- On the exhalation, the practitioner increases the traction of the femur upward out of the hip and creates space between the pelvis and the femur. This is where the concept of using the StretchWave™ is used (described at the start of this chapter) – like the rise and

fall of a wave. The traction up is the rise and movement forward into flexion is the fall.

- Increase ROM in hip flexion is gained by lifting the pelvis and femur upward and moving deeper into hip flexion.
- Turn your hips away from table as you finish.

PNF cue: "Press your leg back into me."

Stretch: Increase hip flexion.

Target tissue – mobilized leg: posterior joint capsule, hamstring and gluteus maximus.

Secondary: Bilateral groin (becomes primary target tissue in hypomobile clients).

Target tissue – immobilized leg: Hip flexors.

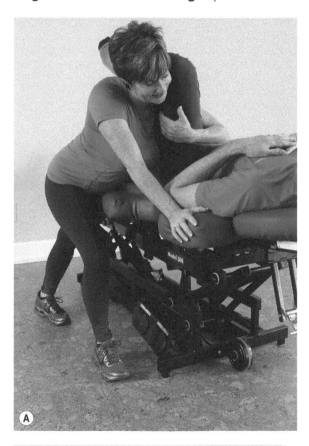

Ⓐ

Figure 5.5a
Hip ROM and PNF

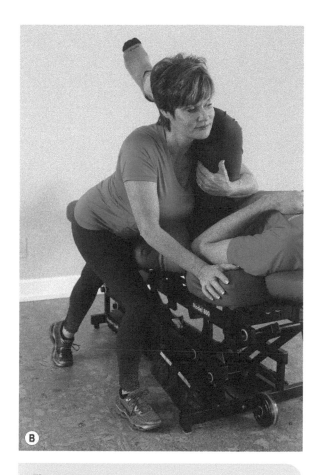

Figure 5.5b
Front view

Repeat: PNF two or more times moving a few degrees out into abduction with each PNF pass for a new angle and different fibers of tissue.

3. Hip/knee flexion with hip abduction – hamstrings, glutei, lumbosacral, hip adductors – SBN, FN, DFN

Goal: To progress from previous stretch by moving into more abduction, slight external rotation; additionally to target the anteromedial joint capsule and tissues in the DFN: short adductors, and proximal attachments of long adductors.

Client position: Same position.

Practitioner:

- From the previous position – your legs are still in a lunge.
- Reach around with your left hand, grab the table for leverage and lean out with your body to move their leg into more abduction.
- Continue moving out to the side (from flexion, adding more abduction) until there is no more resistance in the tissue.

ROM: Progressive increase of hip flexion and abduction with some external rotation.

Traction: Femur up and out of their hip toward their head and then progressing out into abduction with some external rotation.

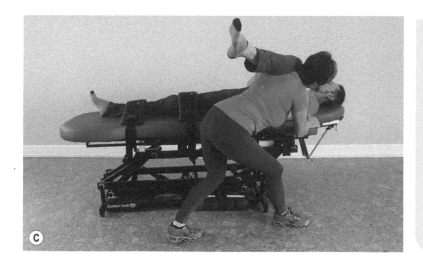

Figure 5.5c
With increased flexion and abduction

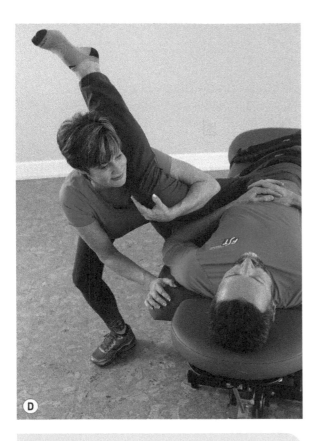

Figure 5.5d
Continue increasing flexion and abduction

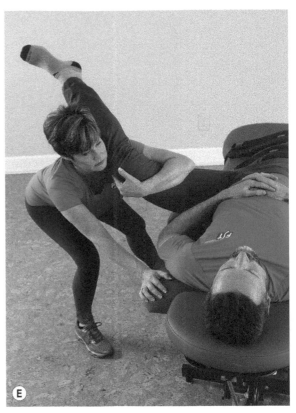

Figure 5.5e
Finish in maximal hip flexion and abduction

Use your shoulder and your body to guide the next position and use the table as leverage to increase your traction.

Remember your legs are creating the traction not your arms.

PNF: Same.

PNF cue: "Press your leg back into me."

Stretch: Increase hip flexion and hip abduction, some external rotation. Finish moving out, down and around to bottom of table. Traction leg out at the bottom corner of the table to finish.

Target: Antero-medial joint capsule, proximal hamstring-adductor interface, bilateral hip adductors.

Repeat: PNF two or more times moving a few degrees out into abduction with each PNF pass for a new angle and different fibers of tissue.

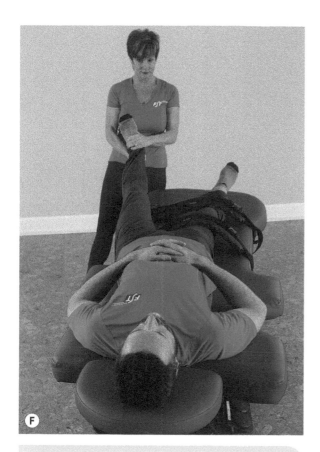

Figure 5.5f
Traction to finish

4. Hip flexion, abduction and external rotation – medial hamstrings and adductors – SBN, FN, DFN

Goal: Target tissues lying within the SBN, FN, DFN: medial hamstrings, adductors.

Client position: Supine with leg opened to side.

Practitioner:

- From the traction at the bottom corner of the table.
- Place their foot in the crease of your hip and support with your leg like it is an extension of the table
- Place your inside hand on their ASIS to stabilize their hip and outside hand on top of their knee, superior to the joint on the distal aspect of the femur.
- Walk up slowly using your hips as you lunge forward to get into the next position.
- To begin with, keep their leg below a 90° horizontal abduction angle.
- Bend forward at the hips, place your heart between your hands.
- **ROM:** Hip flexion and hip abduction.
- **Traction:** Traction the client's femur out by leaning away from the table with your hips.

Hold their foot stable on your body and move their entire leg without losing the angle.

Traction direction is out of the socket first to open the joint – femur away from pelvis.

Traction out then stretch up toward the top of table into deeper flexion.

PNF: Have the client contract glute/hamstring back toward your hip.

PNF cue: "Press your foot back into me."

Stretch: Increase the hip flexion first and then abduction second.

Target tissue: Medial capsule, medial hamstrings, and short hip adductors.

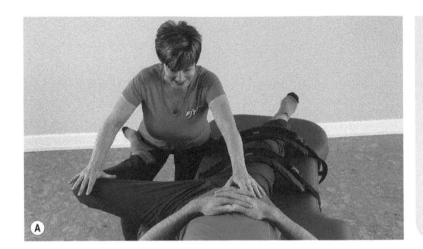

Figure 5.6a
Hip flexion, abduction, ER

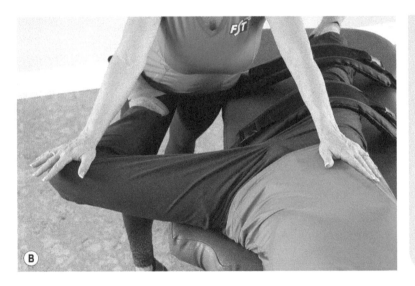

Figure 5.6b
Hand placement – short hip adductor focus

Repeat: PNF one more time.

From the last stretch, we now focus more on the adductors.

5. Hip flexion, abduction, and external rotation – medial hamstrings and short adductors – SBN, FN, DFN

Goal: To target tissues lying within the SBN, FN, DFN: medial hamstrings, short adductors.

Client position: Supine with leg open into abduction.

Practitioner:

- From the previous position, the focus moves to the DFN, FLN, and short adductors.
- Your legs and hands remain in the same position.
- Keep the leg at a 90° angle and use your hips to traction out.
- Drop your body weight down to increase the adduction.
- Remember to use your body and allow the stretch to occur. Don't just push the leg down with your hands.

ROM: Increase ROM by increasing hip abduction and then *flexion*.

Traction: Direction is out of the hip socket to open the joint by moving the femur away from the pelvis.

Use your pecs to spread the tissue open, not just your hands.

PNF: Have the client contract their adductors.

PNF cue: "Press your leg up into my hand toward the ceiling."

Stretch: First increase hip abduction by moving femur down toward the floor. Then increase the hip flexion by moving femur up toward the top of the table.

Rock back and forth to relax the tissue and assess to see what needs more movement.

Repeat: PNF one more time.

- Play with the combination of hip flexion and abduction.
- See if there is a bit more potential in the tissue to release.
- Remember to use your breath and your entire body – not just your hands - when doing the stretch.
- Return the hip back to a closed position by adducting it back to neutral.

6. Low back /thoracic rotation – thoracolumbar fascia, gluteus max, gluteus medius, hip capsule – SBN, SN, FN

Transition: Walk around to the other side of the table and traction leg across the client's body to begin the next stretch.

Low back preparation

Goal: To target tissues lying within the SBN, SN, FN: thoracolumbar fascia, glute max, glute medius, hip capsule.

Target: Thoracolumbar fascia, posterolateral hip capsule, posterior gluteus medius, gluteus maximus.

Client position: Supine with working leg crossed over stationary leg.

Practitioner:

- Cross the client's bent knee and foot over their other leg and place it on the table if possible.
- To begin turn your body toward the client.
- Place your hands on both sides of their knee with one hand above and one below the knee joint.

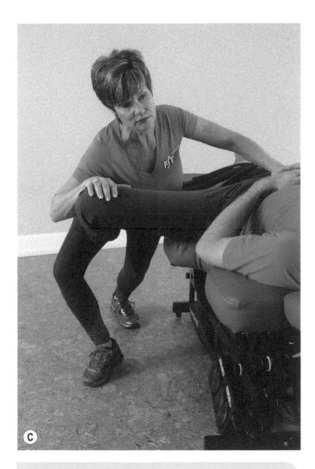

Figure 5.6c
Rock back and forth

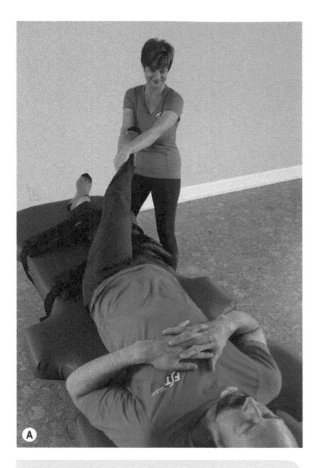

Figure 5.7a
Lateral traction across the body

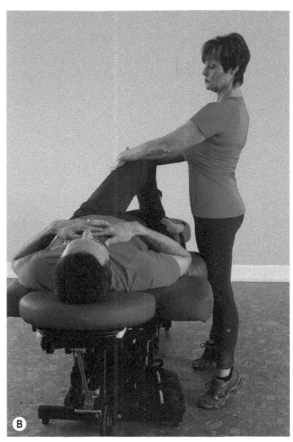

Figure 5.7b
Low back preparation

- Using your body, gently rock their leg back and forth to mobilize and prepare tissues for the stretch.

ROM: Low back thoracic rotation.

Traction: Lift their knee up toward ceiling, then arcing toward you.

Goal: To move the client's femur and pelvis up and over into rotation. Don't just drop the leg down toward the floor.

Practitioner: Use your body to rock back and forth for warm-up – don't just move their leg!

Rise on your toes and then drop down into a squat – do the StretchWave™!

ROM: Increase ROM by increasing hip adduction/internal rotation. Rock back and forth, into and out of ROM.

Traction: Up and over, hip and leg up toward ceiling before down toward table.

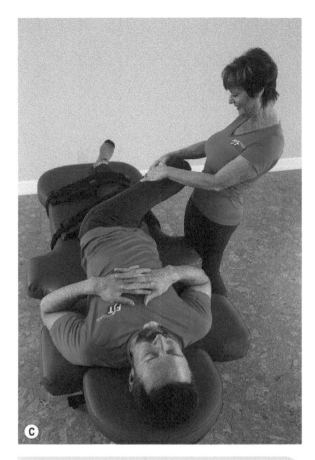

Figure 5.7c
Rocking low back rotation with traction

Practitioner:

- Step down toward the foot of the table and drop your torso across their lower leg.
- Reach across with your inside arm and swing it around to the front of their leg.

Practitioner: Reach out and stabilize hand on the table with outside hand and with inside hand reach across to the opposite side of sacrum lifting pelvis upward.

Practitioner:

- Legs in a lunge position with your torso dropped down onto the client's leg.
- With your inside hand reach all the way to the other side of their sacrum and use your forearm as the fulcrum to cradle their low back. Press into the table with your outside hand for leverage.
- Think of lifting their pelvis up and over.
- Focus on the lift not the rotation.
- Look up to keep focused on lift.

ROM: Increase hip rotation.

Traction: Use your torso to hug your client and your arms to lift their pelvis and femur "up and over".

PNF: Client will try to de-rotate their hips and low back down to the table.

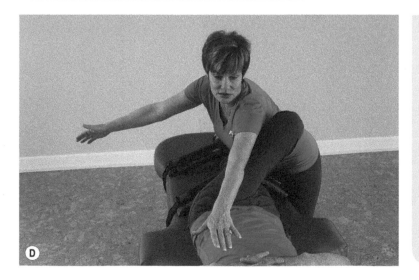

Figure 5.7d
Low back arm reach

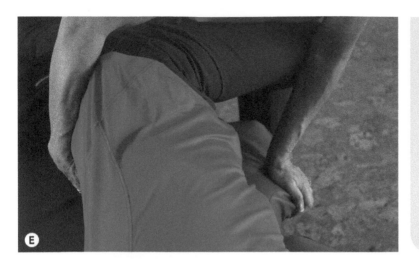

Figure 5.7e
Hand position – both hands shown

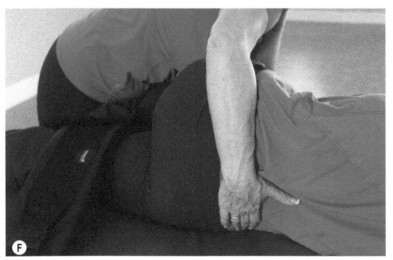

Figure 5.7f
Hand position – back hand shown

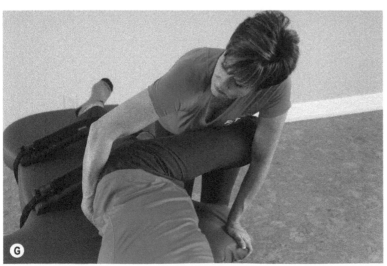

Figure 5.7g
Low back rotation

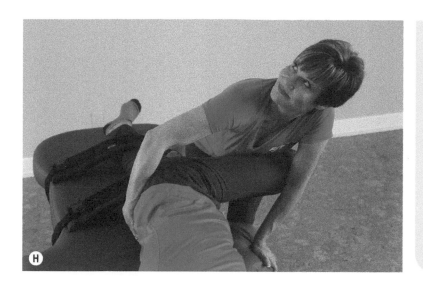

Figure 5.7h
Focus eyes up

PNF cue: "Roll your hips back down to the table."

Stretch: Increase the hip and low back rotation.

Repeat: PNF three or more times.

7. Traction across body

Transition for next move. Traction their left leg across their body.

8. Low back rotation, hip flexion, adduction – thoracolumbar, lateral hamstring – SBN, SN

Goal: To target tissues lying within the SBN, SN: thoracolumbar, lateral hamstring.

Client position: Slight rotation onto side with their left leg across body with bent knee.

Practitioner:

- From the lateral traction across their body, step forward and wrap their leg around your body as you slide into position, hooking in behind their bent knee.
- Your inside hand is lifting their pelvis up and your outside hand is wrapped below around the medial aspect of their femur.
- Keep their knee lifted up and the leg supported and hooked into your body.
- Look up with your eyes to take the focus upward.

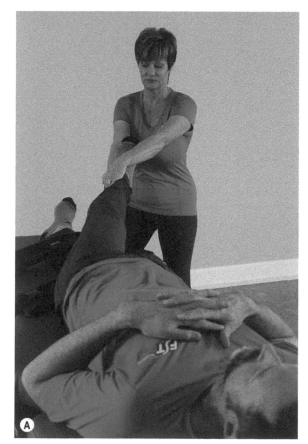

Figure 5.8a
Lateral traction across the body

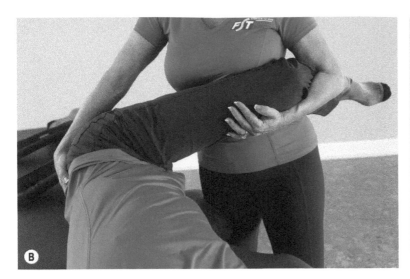

Figure 5.8b
Close up of body position

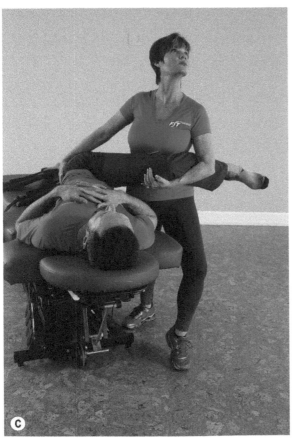

Figure 5.8c
Thoracolumbar posterior hip

ROM: Thoracolumbar rotation and flexion of the femur. Rock back and forth into and out of the range.

Traction: Pelvis up toward the ceiling and into rotation. Femur out of the hip socket (toward upward diagonal).

Lean out with your hips for traction.

PNF: Client contracts hamstring.

PNF cues: "Push your leg back into me."

Stretch: Increase the thoracolumbar rotation and flexion of the femur.

Think of lifting their femur up toward the ceiling and out toward the corner of table.

Repeat: PNF two or more times exploring different angles and fibers.

Signature move

9. "Sack of Buns": thoracolumbar rotation, hip flexion, ER, knee flexion – thoracolumbar, QL, lumbosacral, hip rotators – SFN, SN, DFN

Goal: To target tissues lying within the SFN, SN, DFN: thoracolumbar, QL, lumbosacral, hip rotators.

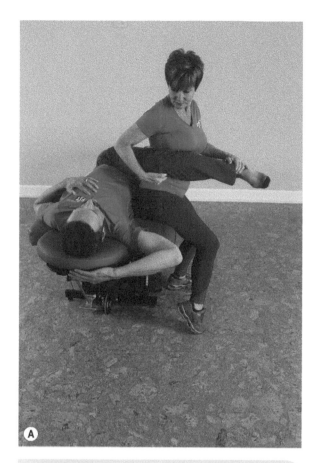

Figure 5.9a
Sack of Buns transition

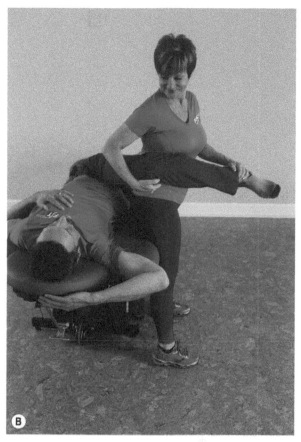

Figure 5.9b
Sack of Buns beginning

To keep the client's knee lifted high and open up the entire area.

Client position: Supine with leg across their body.

Practitioner:

- From the last position, turn around and sit on the table facing away from the client.
- Wrap their leg around your waist or in a place that is comfortable for both of you.
- Your legs are in a wide stance.
- Switch your hand position and wrap your inside hand under the medial aspect of their femur supporting their entire leg by holding it close to your body.

- Your outside hand wraps around the lateral malleolus.
- Stand up and press your own hamstrings back into the table so it won't tip over.
- Lean away from the table with your torso by flexing at the hips.
- Bend your knees and tip your body toward your left foot.
- Press the right side of your pelvis up under their leg and increase your own lateral flexion by leaning away from the client. Keep at least one leg pressing against table.

ROM: External rotation of their femur and lower leg.

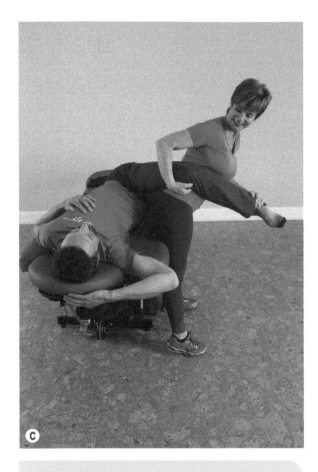

Figure 5.9c
Sack of Buns stretch

Traction: Traction is up toward the ceiling and the femur lifted out of the hip socket.

PNF:

Action 1: Client contracts to pull their femur into internal rotation.

Action 2: Client contracts entire leg into internal rotation.

PNF cues: Cue 1: "Pull your knee down to the floor." **Cue 2:** "Press your ankle up into my hand."

Stretch: Increase stretch by increasing their external rotation of the femur by lifting it up and pressing downward on the lateral malleolus.

Play with the amount of traction and variety of angles.

Get your front hip up and under their leg. Bend forward from the hips – and away!

Repeat: PNF two or more times.

From Sack of Buns, traction leg out for transition to prepare for glutes series.

Traction leg out across their body.

10. Hip flexion, external rotation, adduction, knee flexed 45° – gluteus medius, piriformis – LN, SN

Goal: To target tissues lying within the LN, SN: gluteus medius, piriformis.

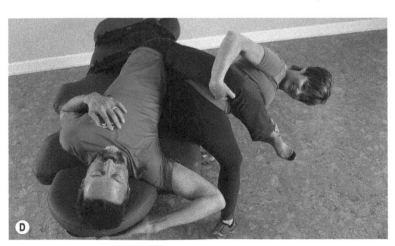

Figure 5.9d
Sack of Buns max

Practitioner:

- Preparation and beginning position: start at the bottom of the table and walk their leg up into position.
- Allow their knee to bend, supporting their foot, and moving their leg toward them.
- Place their foot in the crease of your outside hip or find a comfortable position for both of you.
- Keep their foot lower than their knee (i.e. toward floor not ceiling).
- Lean your body back to get into the position and stand up straight.
- Lift up onto the balls of your feet to lift the femur upward and create traction
- Place your inside hand on the back of their knee and the other hand on the lateral ankle. Place their ankle in the crease of your hip for support and comfort.
- Lean gently forward to find their R1
- Keep their foot in the crease of your hip and below their knee.

TIP

Use your body and legs to increase the traction and the stretch – as opposed to using more pressure with your hands. The focus is on their ankle with gentle pressure down toward the floor, not on the knee.

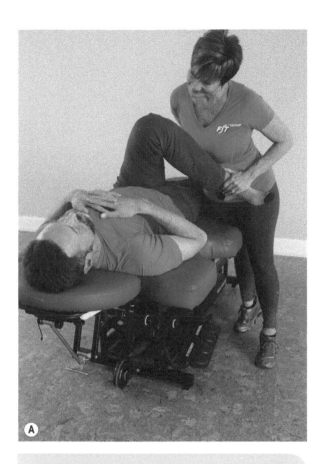

Figure 5.10a
Gluteus medius beginning

Client position: Supine with left leg bent across chest.

Try to have their knee toward the center of their chest if possible.

ROM: Hip flexion and adduction.

Traction: Traction their hip upward as you move their bent knee down toward the center of their chest.

PNF: Get the client to contract the hip back into extension.

PNF cues: "Push your knee back into my hand."

Stretch: Increase hip flexion and adduction. Bring their entire leg down toward chest.

With each PNF pass, move a few degrees across the fan of their hip.

Repeat: PNF two or more times.

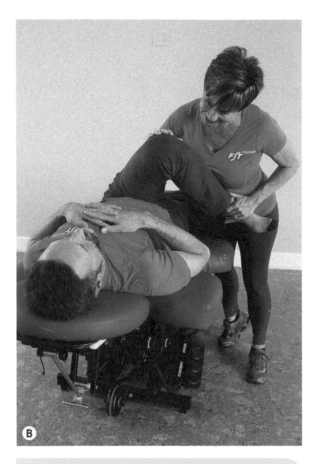

Figure 5.10b
Gluteus medius stretch

Alternate hand position

This is an alternate hand position, especially if there is pinching in the front of the client's hip.

- Slide your hand completely under the pelvis and lift it up off the table into a posterior tilt.
- Try to put more emphasis on their foot – pressing downward.
- Remember the focus is on the ankle, not the knee.
- From the stretch, continue the motion by swooping their knee down toward their opposite shoulder.
- Drop your body weight down on to their leg to keep the stretch going.
- Don't just push with your hands.
- Move very slowly as you continue down and around in a big circular movement.
- Keep swooping.
- Release their leg from the swoop and let it straighten out as you walk backwards.
- Walk down to the bottom corner of the table.
- Finish with lateral traction across their body.

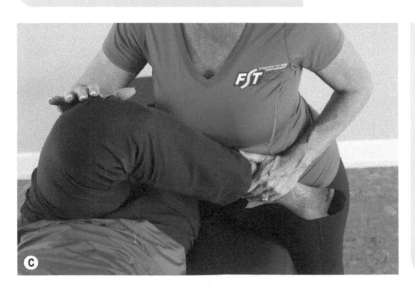

Figure 5.10c
Hand position

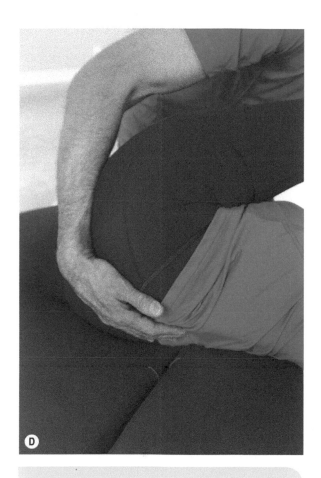

Figure 5.10d
Alternative hand position for gluteus medius

11. Hip flexion, adduction, external rotation, knee flexed 90° – hip extensors, gluteus maximus – FN

Posterior fibers of the hip

TIP

Reach your arm out and use your body to float up and move into a deeper stretch.

Signature move

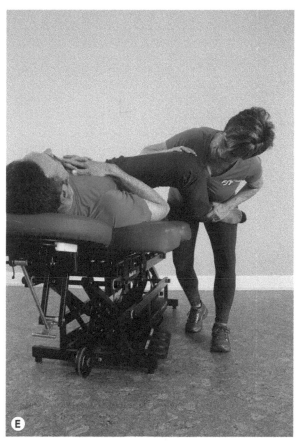

Figure 5.10e
Glute swoop

Goal: Target tissues lying within the FN: posterior fibers of gluteus maximus. Getting the femur toward their chest is the first goal and external rotation is the second goal.

Target all of the fibers in the fan of the hip.

Client position: Supine with their leg crossed over their body at a 90° angle.

Practitioner:

- From the previous position of lateral traction at the end of the table, walk back slowly into the new position.
- Bend their leg into a 90° angle, if possible, in relation to the femur and the lower leg bones.
- Aim their left knee to the same (left) shoulder to start.
- Place the heel of their foot in the space between your anterior deltoid and pectoralis major on shoulder or wherever it works best for both of you.
- Place one hand on lateral left knee and the other hand in front of their right ankle to hold it secure.

ROM: Hip flexion.

Traction: Lift the femur up and out of the hip socket. Traction "up" (StretchWave™ toward their head).

Place their foot on your shoulder to increase traction upward. Use your body rather than your hands to traction their leg up.

PNF: Client contracts their bent leg back into extension.

PNF cues: "Push your knee back into my hand."

Stretch: Increase hip flexion.

Getting the femur toward their chest is the first goal; rotation is the second goal.

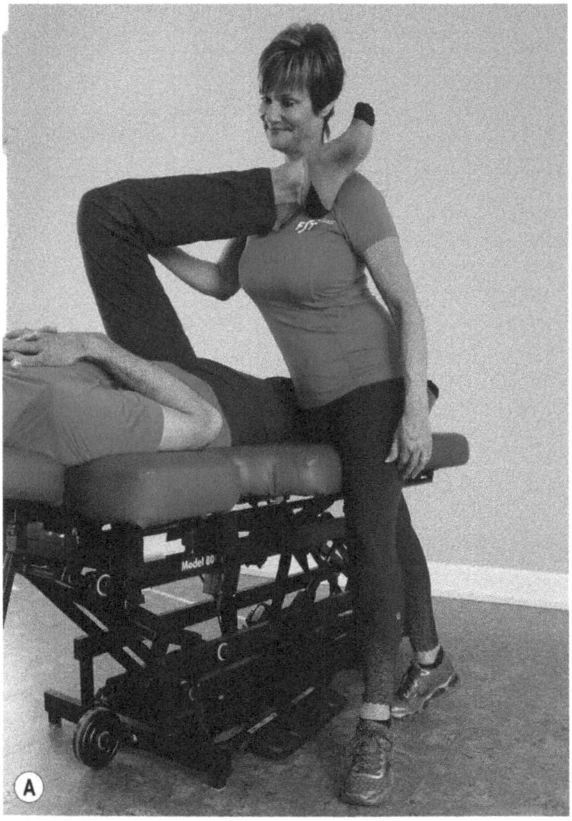

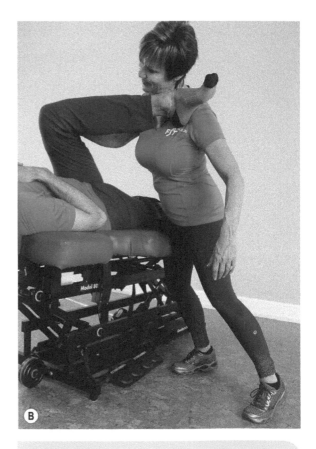

Figure 5.11a
Glute maximus beginning

Figure 5.11b
Glute maximus stretch

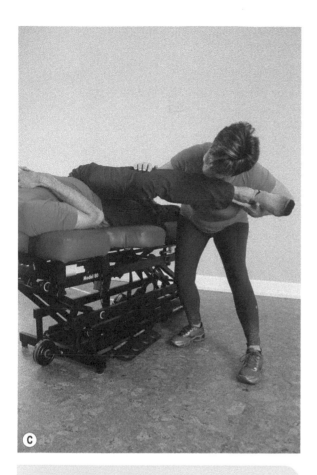

- Move very slowly as you continue down and around in a big circular movement.
- Keep swooping around.
- Release their leg from the swoop and let it straighten out as you walk backwards.
- Walk down to the bottom corner of the table.
- Finish with lateral traction across their body.

C. Range of Motion Evaluation, Warm-up and FST PNF Stretch – Straight Leg and Multiple Joints

Multiple plane soft tissue ROM evaluation and stretch

- Move only to R1 for warm-up.
- Exhale into all ROM increases.
- Use gentle StretchWave™ movements throughout.
- Move in 3–5° increments as you assess tissue; checking the ROM at each range moving in the circle, like a stopwatch smoothly ticking.

From the bent leg series, continue working with their left leg to complete the lines.

Figure 5.11c
Glute swoop

Targeting all of the fiber of the posterior hip.

With each PNF pass, move a few degrees across the fan of their hip.

Repeat: PNF two or more times. Explore all of the angles and fibers.

- From the stretch, continue the motion by swooping their knee down toward their opposite shoulder.
- Drop your body weight down onto their leg to keep the stretch going – don't just push with your hands.

1. Hip flexion, knee extension – hamstrings – SBN, SN

TIP

Use soft hands – no gripping, "If you are squeezing, you aren't pleasing!" Use their heel for the traction upward.

Goal: To target tissues lying within the SBN, SN: hamstrings.

Client position: Supine with their extended leg up in hip flexion.

Practitioner:

- Your legs are in a lunge position with your outside leg forward and your inside leg back.
- Place your outside hand on the back of their heel and use it as the anchor point to traction the femur out of the joint and into the ROM.

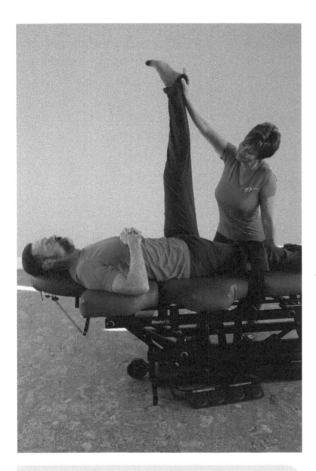

Figure 5.12
Hip flexion, knee extension – sagittal direction

- Engage your lat for stability and strength.
- Place your inside hand on the table for leverage.
- Think about getting underneath their leg to lift it upward.

ROM: Hip flexion

Traction: Traction "up and out" (out of the socket and toward their head)

PNF: Client contracts their hamstrings into extension.

PNF cues: "Press your leg back into me."

Stretch: Increase hip flexion.

Repeat: PNF two or more times.

2. Hip flexion, abduction, knee extension – medial hamstrings – DFN, SBN, SN

Increase ROM and stretch by increasing hip flexion and abduction. Think of the client's leg floating smoothly out to the side and then down and around to the bottom of the table.

Goal: To target tissues lying within the SBN, FN, DFN: hamstrings and adductors.

Continue from last position by increasing the ROM as their leg moves out and around to the side.

Client position: Supine with their leg in flexion.

Practitioner:

- Your leg and outside hand position remains the same until their leg moves out into abduction.
- Move your outside hand and place it behind their knee for support.
- Use your body to maintain the traction and increase abduction.

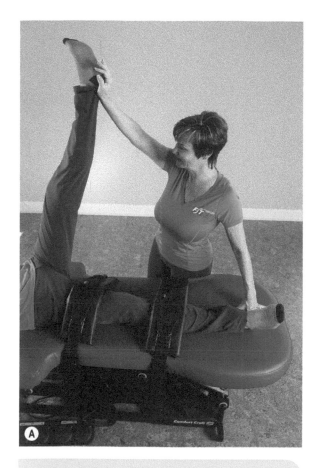

Figure 5.13a
Hip flexion

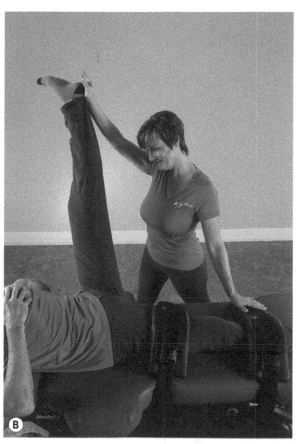

Figure 5.13b
Hip flexion and abduction

ROM: Hip flexion and abduction.

Traction: Traction up, out and open (out of socket, toward their head and out to side).

PNF: Client contracts their hamstrings into extension and adductors in slight adduction.

PNF cues: "Press your leg back in to me."

Stretch: Increasing hip flexion and abduction.

Repeat: PNF two or more times.

Traction their leg in a slightly more open abducted position.

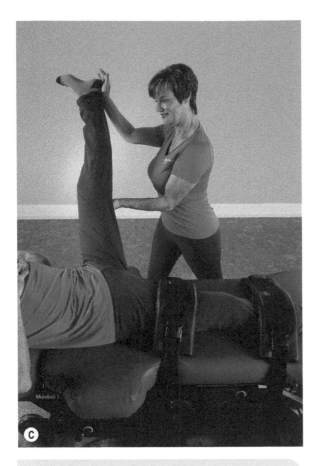

Figure 5.13c
Abduction and hip flexion, ER

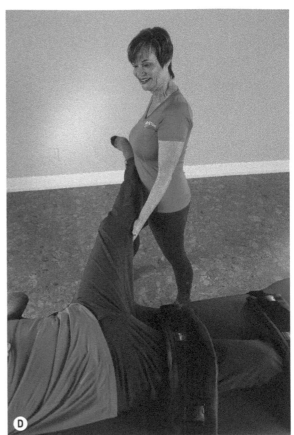

Figure 5.13d
Medial hamstring focus

3. Hip flexion, abduction, knee extension – medial hamstring focus – SBN, SN, FN, DFN

Goal: To target tissues lying within the SBN, SN, FN, DFN and hip flexion: medial hamstrings.

Client position: Supine with outside leg in hip flexion and abduction.

Practitioner:

- Place their leg across your hips.
- Hook their heel on the outside of your hip, hugging it against you with your outside hand.

- Place your other hand behind their knee for support.

ROM: Hip flexion (move their leg toward the top of the table).

Hip abduction (down toward the floor).

Traction: Out of the hip socket away from their pelvis.

Traction by leaning your body away from the table – use your hips! Increase the traction by lunging out to the side.

PNF: Client contracts hamstrings

PNF cue: "Press your leg back into me."

Stretch: Hip flexion and abduction

Repeat: PNF two or more times.

4. Hip flexion, abduction, knee extension – long adductors focus – SBN, FN, SN, DFN

Goal: To target tissues lying within the SBN, FN, SN, DFN: long adductors.

Client position: Supine with leg in hip flexion and abduction.

Practitioner: From last position; keep leg across your hips.

Change the hand position from last stretch. Move your hand to top of their leg on the medial side of their distal femur and medial ankle.

Use your hips to traction by lunging out to side. Slide their leg down your leg with your hands. Or bend your knees to lower their leg.

Take care of your back – don't bend over too much!

ROM: Hip flexion and abduction.

Traction: Out of the hip socket to the side and down toward the floor.

PNF: Client contracts their adductors.

PNF cue: "Press your entire leg up to the ceiling."

Stretch: Increase abduction by sliding their leg down your leg toward floor.

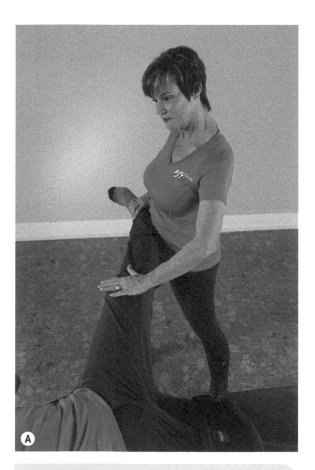

Figure 5.14a
Adductor focus

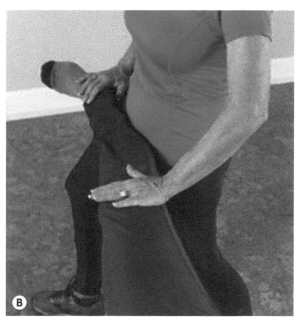

Figure 5.14b
Adductor focus – close up

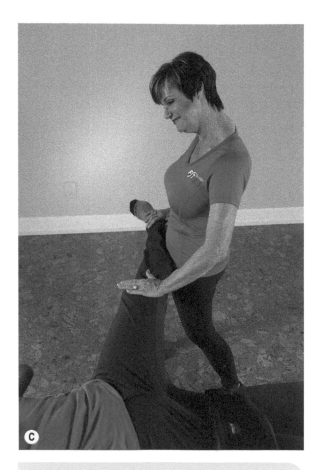

Figure 5.14c
Increased adductor focus

Repeat: PNF two or more times.

Play with alternating between the angles and different fibers of the tissues here.

5. Hip flexion, abduction, knee extension – hamstrings and long adductors combination – SBN, FN, SN, DFN

Goal: To target tissues lying within the SBN, FN, SN, DFN: hamstrings and long adductors.

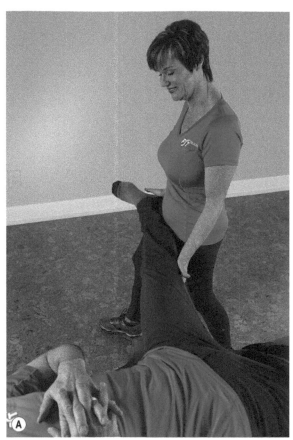

Figure 5.15a
Practitioner position finds interface between medial hamstrings and adductors

Client position: Supine with leg in hip flexion and abduction.

Practitioner:

- From the previous position, release the stretch and reduce ROM.
- The practitioner now brings a combination of movement of hip flexion and adduction.

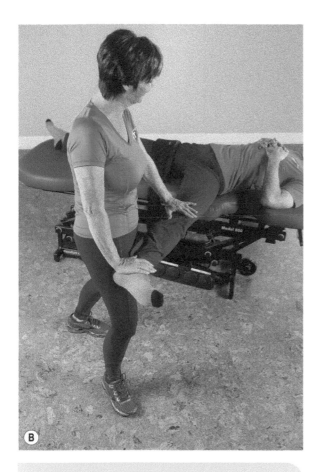

(B)

Figure 5.15b
PNF combination of medial hamstring and adductors

- Reposition the client's leg up across your hips again.
- Create traction by using your hips to lean away from the table.
- Move your hands back to more a medial aspect of their femur again, but still have some contact with the adductors.
- Hold their heel across your hip for support.

ROM: Hip flexion and abduction.

Traction: Out of the hip socket to the side, down toward the floor, and then up into flexion. Use your entire body to traction by leaning away from the table.

PNF: Client contracts both their hamstring and adductor at the same time.

PNF cue: "Press your leg back into me and upward toward ceiling."

Stretch:

- Increase hip flexion and abduction.
- Increase stretch by moving femur away from the pelvis, down toward the floor, and then up toward the top of the table.
- Play with alternating between the angles and different fibers of the tissues.

Repeat: PNF two or more times.

Use traction to transition to lateral aspect of the hamstrings on the other side of the table.

6. Hip flexion, adduction, internal rotation with lumbar rotation – low back, glutes, IT band, fibularis – SBN, LN

Goal: Target tissues lying within the SBN, LN: low back, glutes, IT band, fibularis.

Client position: Partial side lying with the working leg adducted across their stationary leg.

Practitioner:

- Sit on the table if you need to for position.
- Drop your weight down and lean away to find ROM and increase traction.
- Drop the client's leg toward the floor with your hands placed on the outside of the knee and above their ankle.

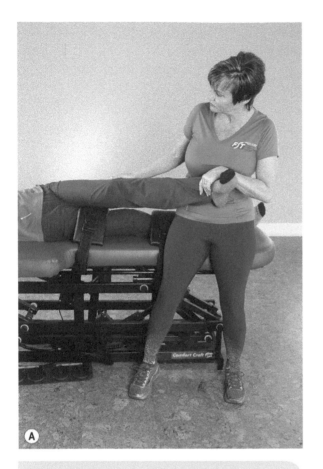

(A)

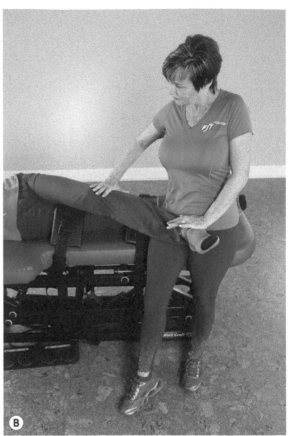

(B)

Figure 5.16a
Lateral traction and out to corner and down toward floor

Figure 5.16b
Lateral net and lateral hamstring down to the floor

ROM: Adduction, internal rotation and hip flexion with lumbar rotation.

Traction: Traction leg out (of hip socket), away from the table and down toward the floor.

PNF: Client contracts the lateral aspect of the hip and leg up into abduction.

PNF cues: "Press your entire leg up toward the ceiling."

Stretch: Increase adduction, internal rotation and hip flexion with lumbar rotation.

Repeat: PNF two or more times.

If you were sitting on the table, stand up and traction leg across client's body before moving into the next stretch.

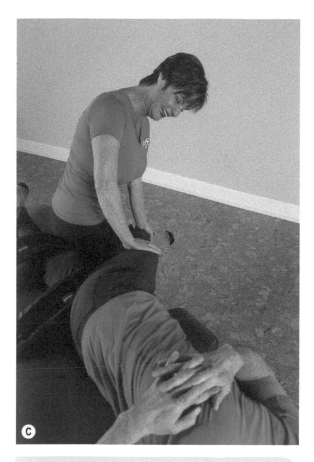

Figure 5.16c
Hand position top

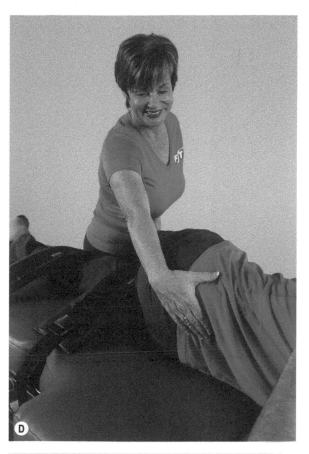

Figure 5.16d
Hand position with SI support

7. Hip flexion, adduction, knee extension, lumbar rotation – low back, lateral hamstrings, glutes, IT band, fibularis – LN, SN, SBN

Goal: To target tissues lying within the SN, SBN: low back, glutes, IT band, fibularis.

Client position: Supine to partial side lying with their leg adducted across their body.

Practitioner:

- From the previous position, step out to the side away from the table.

- Place the client's leg across your hip and hook their heel on the outside for support and traction.

- Place your outside hand on the top their ankle and hold it close to your body. The inside hand behind their knee for support.

ROM: Hip flexion with lumbar rotation and adduction.

Traction: Out of the hip socket and up toward the top of the table. Use your body to move their leg into increased ROM and stretch.

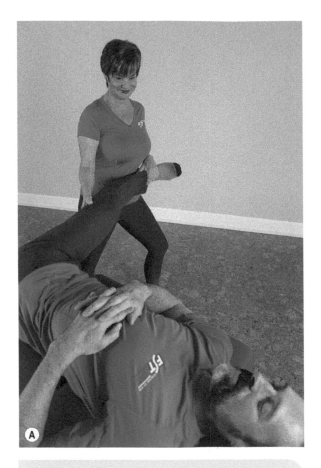

Figure 5.17a
Lateral traction

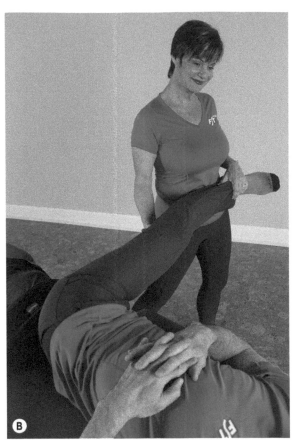

Figure 5.17b
Mid-position

PNF: Client contracts their hamstring.

PNF cue: "Press your leg back into my body."

Stretch: Increase hip flexion with lumbar rotation and adduction.

Repeat: PNF two or more times.

Increase the stretch by increasing hip flexion toward the top of the table on a diagonal and up.

8. Hip flexion, adduction, internal rotation with lumbar rotation – low back, glutes, IT band, fibularis – lateral hamstrings, high position – SN, SBN

Goal: To target tissues lying within the SN, SBN and lateral hamstrings in a new angle.

Client position: Supine.

Practitioner: From the previous position, lift the client's leg higher toward to the ceiling. Place

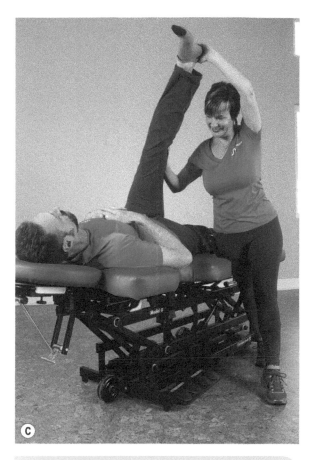

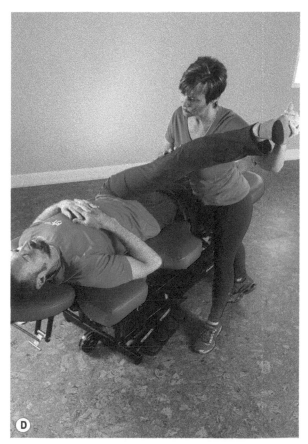

Figure 5.17c
High position 1 focus on lateral hamstring, SN, SBN

Figure 5.17d
High position 2 continue arc across body

your hands on the heel and on the back of their hamstring.

Traction: Out of the hip socket and up to the diagonal, top corner of table toward opposite shoulder.

ROM: Hip flexion with lumbar rotation and adduction.

Traction: Out and up.

PNF: Client contracts their hamstring.

PNF cues: "Press your leg back to me."

Stretch: Increase hip flexion with lumbar rotation and adduction. Leg is up and across on the diagonal.

Repeat: PNF two or more times.

> **NOTE**
> The client's knee should not be bent past 90°
> for the following stretches 2, 3, or 4 or it will
> become a quad stretch too soon.

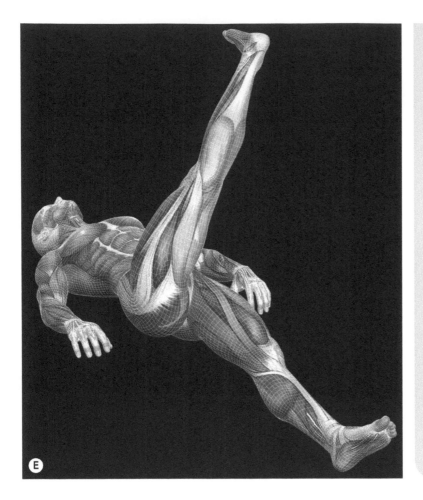

E

Figure 5.17e
Target tissues within
Superficial Back Net

D. Range of Motion Evaluation, Warm-up, and FST PNF Stretch

1. Pelvic external rotation – iliacus and psoas – DFN

Goal: To target tissues lying within the DFN: proximal iliacus and distal psoas increase external rotation of the pelvic bone.

Client position: Lying on their side with top leg in extended hip neutral and bottom leg up into partial hip and knee flexion. Make sure their hips remain stacked on top on each other and their arms are resting comfortably.

Practitioner:

- Turn your body toward the foot of the table and sit on the edge, facing away from the client. Place your inside leg on the table and your outside foot firmly planted on the floor.
- Support their lower back with your inside hip.
- Move your body toward the client to get into position.

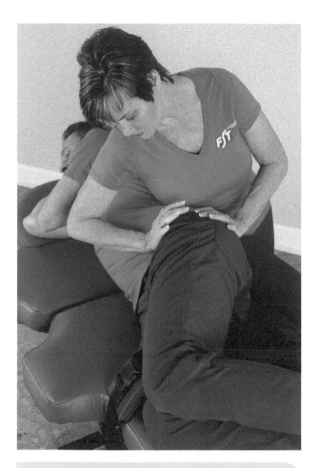

Figure 5.18
Pelvic rocking into external rotation

- Place inside hand on the front of their ASIS and the other hand on the back of the PSIS. Find the best position for your own body.
- Cup their pelvis between your hands.
- Move in a gentle rocking motion back and forth. It is a small movement.

ROM: External rotation of the pelvic bone to aid hip extension.

Traction: Lift the front of their pelvis up toward the ceiling. PNF: Client contracts their iliacus and psoas into your front hand.

PNF cue: "Roll your abdominals and hip down to the table."

Stretch:

- Increase external rotation of the pelvic bone, target iliacus.
- Re-check passive ROM.

Repeat: PNF two or more times.

> **NOTE**
> The client's knee should not be bent past 90° for the following stretches 2, 3, or 4 or it will become a quad stretch too soon.

2. Hip extension – hip flexors – SFN, DFN, FN, SN, LN

Goal: To target tissues lying within the SFN, DFN, FN, SN, LN: proximal attachments of hip flexors.

To increase hip extension.

Client position: Lying on their side with top leg in hip extension, slight knee flexion and bottom leg up into hip flexion and bent at the knee. Make sure their shoulders and hips remain stacked on top on each other and their arms are resting comfortably.

Practitioner:

- From the previous position, stand up and turn around to face the client.
- Step away from the table with your outside foot.
- Place their lower leg across your body and hook the client's foot on your outside hip or wherever it feels the most comfortable.
- Wrap your outside hand around the bottom of their foot and hold it close to your body.
- Place your inside hand on their femur above their knee for support.
- Hug their foot into your body and lean away to traction.
- Move back and forth into and out of extension.
- Dance with them to mobilize various angles before stretching.

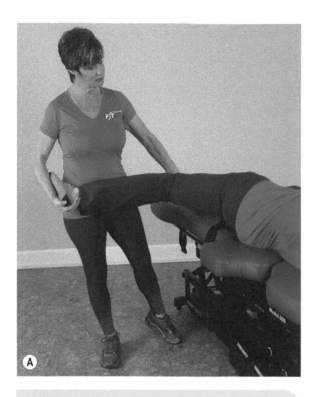

Figure 5.19a
Hip extension for hip flexor proximal attachments

ROM: Hip extension.

Traction: Move the client's femur into extension. Use your whole body to move their leg.

PNF: Client rolls their body down to the table and contracts their hip flexors.

PNF cue: *From origin* "Roll your abs and hip down to the table." *From insertion*: "Pull your knee toward your other leg." *Origin and insertion PNF combo*: "Roll and pull."

Stretch: Increase hip extension.

Repeat: PNF two or more times.

TIP

Make sure the placement of the client's foot is comfortable and feels secure for both of you.

NOTE
Remember: the placement may be a little different for each client. If the position is not correct their ankle may feel caught. Use your lats and drop your body weight down for additional leverage.

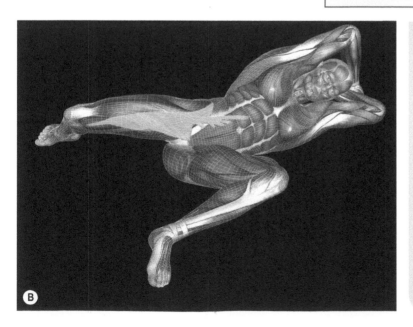

Figure 5.19b
Target tissues primarily in the Deep Front Net

3. Hip extension, adduction – hip flexors and abductors – SFN, DFN, FN, SN, LN

Goal: To target tissues lying within the SFN, DFN, FN, SN, FN: lateral fibers of hip flexors and abductors.

Increased hip extension and hip adduction.

Client position: Lying on their side with top leg in hip extension, slight knee flexion and bottom leg up into hip flexion and bent at the knee. Make sure their hips and shoulders remain stacked on top on each other and that their arms are resting comfortably.

Practitioner:

- From the last position, move closer in and toward the table again.
- Drop the client's lower leg down across your thigh or into whatever position is comfortable for both of you.

Practitioner's hand position:

- Hinge forward at the hips and place your chest over the top of their femur.
- Bend your knees and lower your entire body to change the angle of the leg.
- Wrap your both arms around their femur and hug their leg into your body.

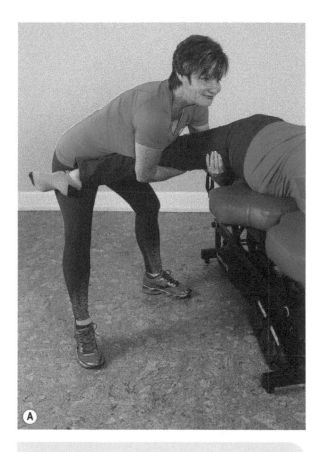

Figure 5.20a
Hip extension for anterior and lateral fibers of hip flexors

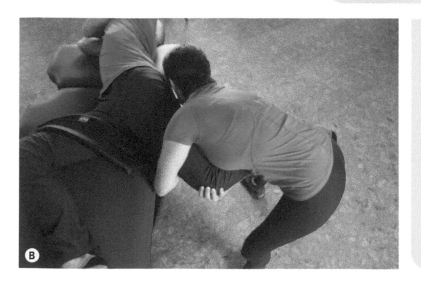

Figure 5.20b
Hip extension focused on lateral fibers

- Support the femur with one hand and the knee with the other hand.
- Lean your hips away from the table for the traction.
- Use your body weight to increase the stretch by dropping your weight gently down onto client's leg.
- Be aware of keeping their femur and lower leg in proper alignment for the safety of the knee, especially the medial aspect.
- The client's knee should not be bent past 90° or it will become a quad stretch too soon, which comes later.

ROM: Hip extension and adduction.

Traction: Femur out of hip socket. Think of tractioning all of the tissue as you move it into extension and adduction.

PNF: Client contracts lateral aspect of upper leg and hip.

PNF cue: "Lift your leg up into me," (toward the ceiling).

Stretch: Increase hip extension and adduction.

Repeat: PNF two or more times.

4. Hip extension – hip flexors – fascial component – SFN, DFN, FN, SN

Goal: To target tissues lying within the SFN, DFN, FN, SN: entire hip flexors complex with all the fascial components.

To increase hip extension to its fullest potential using more traction!

Client position: Lying on their side with top leg in hip extension, slight knee flexion and bottom leg up into hip flexion and bent at the knee. Arms resting comfortably.

Practitioner:

- From the previous position, stand up and lunge away from the table with your outside foot.

- Hook their foot on your outside hip, hold their heel in your hand.
- Place your inside hand on their femur above their knee for support.
- Allow knee to just rest in your palm.
- Keep their foot secured into your body and lean away to traction.
- Lean away with your body to increase the stretch.

ROM: hip extension.

Traction: Out – moving the femur into extension. Increase the traction by leaning away with your body more.

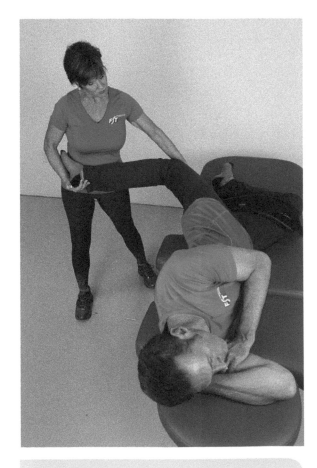

Figure 5.21
Increased hip extension

PNF: Client contracts entire hip flexor complex.

PNF cue: "Pull your entire leg across your body."

Stretch: Increase hip extension. Play with the angles.

Repeat: PNF two or more times.

5. Hip extension, knee flexion – quadriceps focus – SFN, DFN, FN, SN

> **NOTE**
> It is very important to move slowly and gently into knee flexion.

Goal: To target SFN, DFN, FN, SN, hip flexors and quads.

To increase hip extension and knee flexion.

Client position: Lying on their side with top leg in hip extension, knee flexion about 90° and bottom leg up into hip flexion and bent at the knee. Arms resting comfortably.

Practitioner:

- From last position, reduce the hip extension a bit and slowly increase the knee flexion.
- Square your hips off to face the table and move your body closer to the top of table.
- Increase the stretch.
- You can move back and forth from the hip extension to the knee flexion.
- Swing your hips closer to into the top of table to increase knee flexion.
- You can intensify the stretch by combining the hip and knee flexion, but be gentle as this is a very deep stretch.

ROM: Hip extension and knee flexion

Traction: Femur out of the hip socket.

PNF: Client contracts their quadriceps by extending knee.

PNF cue: "Kick me!" We find this is a better cue than "Extend your knee!"

Stretch: Hip extension and knee flexion.

Slowly bend their knee toward glutes (increase knee flexion)

Repeat: PNF two or more times. Play with the angles.

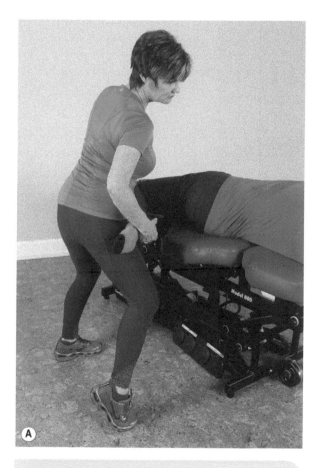

Figure 5.22a
Increase knee flexion

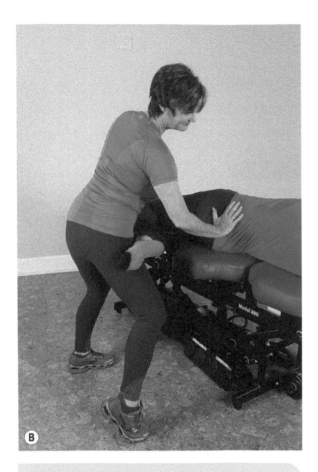

Figure 5.22b
Alternate hand position to support their lower back

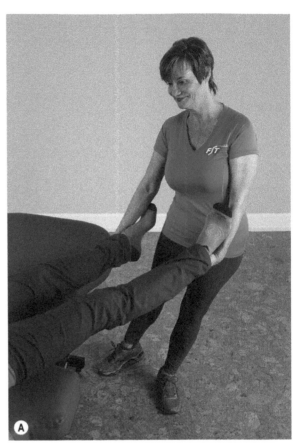

Figure 5.23a
Lateral Net for the left side

Repeat hip flexor and quad series on the other side or repeat B through E on other leg, depending on whole or partial sequence.

E. Lateral Net

1. Low back side bend from below – fascia from fibularis (peroneals) to QL – LN, SN

Goal: To target the tissues lying within the LN, SN: lateral hip and torso, fascia from fibularis (peroneals) to QL.

Increase lateral flexion.

Client position: Supine with arms at their side.

Practitioner:

- Lifts both of client's legs for passive extension with traction at 10–20°.
- Hold both of their heels in the palms of your hands and gently wrap your fingers around their heels.
- Engage your core and bend your knees slightly.
- Double leg traction to begin.

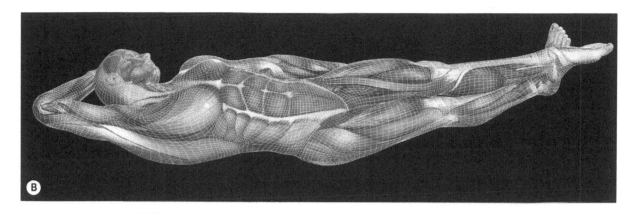

Figure 5.23b Target tissues within the Lateral Net

ROM: Then move slowly to your left side until the client's movement stops at R1.

Traction: Lean back with your body, staying relaxed.

Practitioner:

- Continuing on from double leg traction ...
- Once their legs clear the table as you move farther to the side, place the client's lateral malleolus (the bottom leg) on your femur or hip with your inside hand securing it to your body.
- Lift their right leg higher, cradle their heel close into your body with your outside hand.
- Use your inside hand for the PNF cue on the outside of the left leg.
- Lean your torso back as you press your hips into a posterior tilt to increase the stretch.

ROM: Increase ROM by increasing lateral flexion.

Traction: Lean away.

PNF: Client contracts the lateral aspect of the left leg.

PNF cue: "Press your leg back into me."

Stretch: Increase their lateral flexion.

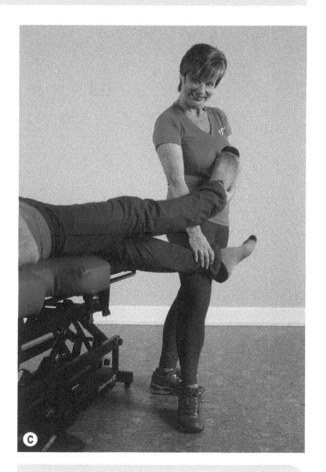

Figure 5.23c
Lateral Net (legs crossed)

Practitioner:

- From the last position, shift your body weight back onto your heels to reduce the tissue tension and use your inside hand to slide their left leg down your body to increase the stretch and target different fibers.
- Continue to lunge as you slide their leg down your quad and lean back slightly to increase the stretch.

Traction: Keep tractioning out as you move. Think of the traction as if you are moving together in an arc away from the table and then up toward the top of the table.

Use your body and not your arms to feel the tissue as you lean away from the table.

PNF: Client contracts the lateral aspect of the left leg.

PNF cue: "Press your leg back into me."

Stretch: Increase their lateral flexion (slide their leg down toward floor).

Repeat: PNF two or more times.

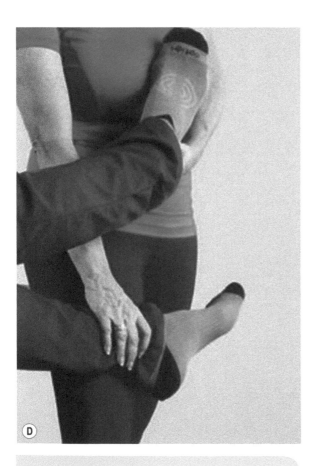

Figure 5.23d
Lateral Net close up

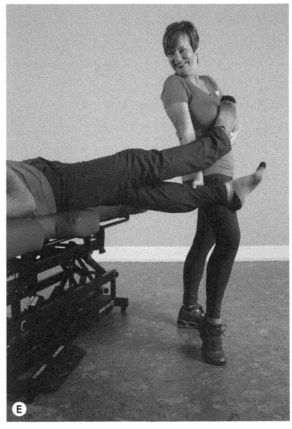

Figure 5.23e
Lateral Net

F. Repeat Entire Series on the Right Leg B through D.

Now repeat Lateral Net to the right side to finish.

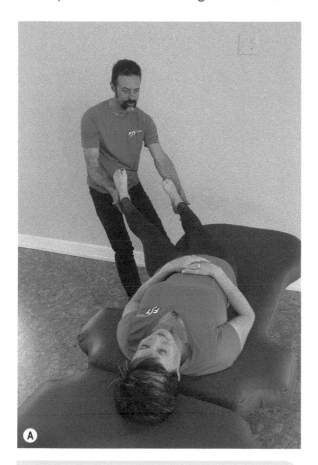

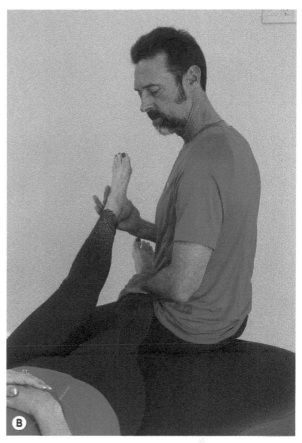

Figure 5.24b
Lateral Net moving to the right. For a very restricted client, the practitioner can sit on the table

Figure 5.24a
Lateral Net moving to the right

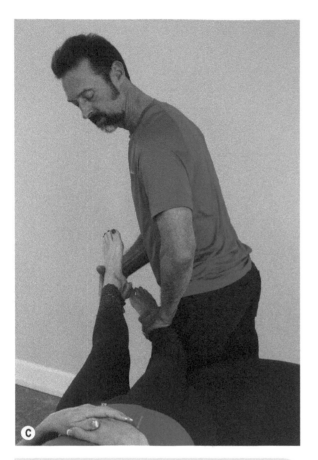

Figure 5.24c
Stand up

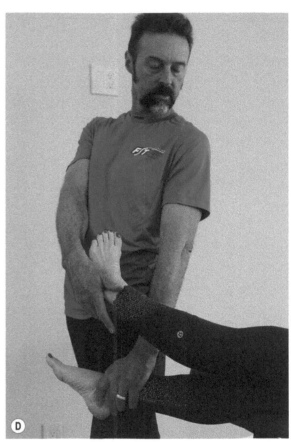

Figure 5.24d
Stretch

G. Pelvic Stabilization and Sacral Set

Essential movement to finish all table sequences (long or short).

1. Abductor contractions

Goal: To give client pelvic stability and proprioceptive grounding after the lower body work on the table.

Client position: Supine, with their knees together and bent, both feet flat on the table about a foot away from hips.

Practitioner: Can be up on top of table straddling client or on the floor.

Hands can be placed outside the knees if there is any question of knee injury or instability.

PNF: They abduct their legs against your total 100% resistance three times.

PNF Cue: "Open your knees."

2. Adductor contractions

Practitioner: Right arm in between the client's legs.

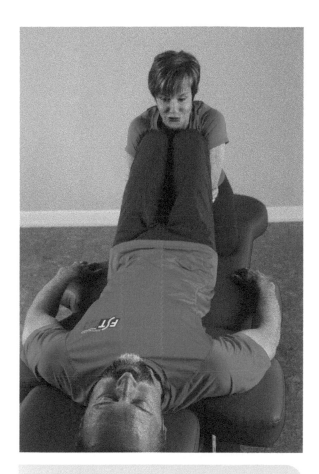

Figure 5.25
Pelvic stabilization

Client position: They give a 100% contraction.

PNF: "Squeeze your knees into me."

Practitioner: Left arm in between the client's legs.

Client position: They give a 100% contraction.

PNF: "Squeeze again."

Practitioner: Both arms between their legs.

Client position: They give a 100% contraction.

PNF: "Squeeze your knees into me one more time."

3. Sacral set

Goal: To ensure sacrum/SI joints are positioned and stabilized back to neutral position.

Client position: Same position.

Practitioner:

- Press knees straight downward into table through the femurs at an angle of 45° to reset the sacrum to a neutral position.
- Hands should be straight underneath your body with fingertips facing out. They are placed on the client's femurs not on their kneecaps.
- Lock your elbows and drive all of your weight straight down through their femurs.

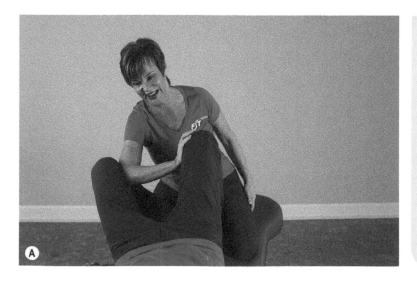

Figure 5.26a
Right arm in

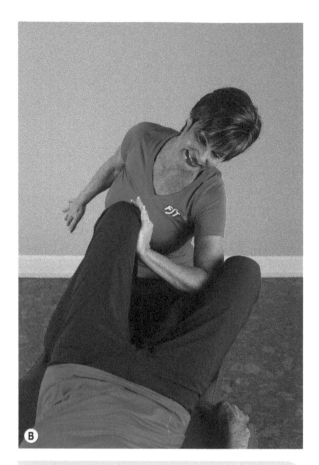

Figure 5.26b
Left arm in

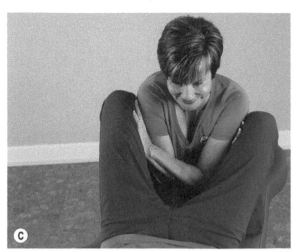

Figure 5.26c
Both arms in

- Tuck your elbows into your torso for extra support.
- Ask if the pressure feels evenly distributed.
- Stay there for a minute and then gently pulse downward.
- Tell your client, "Relax and breathe."

Optional position

Practitioner:

Holds on to both sides of the table and pulls upward using their pecs to drive the femur's back into the hip sockets.

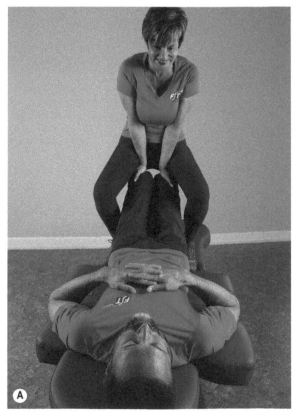

Figure 5.27a
Sacral set front view

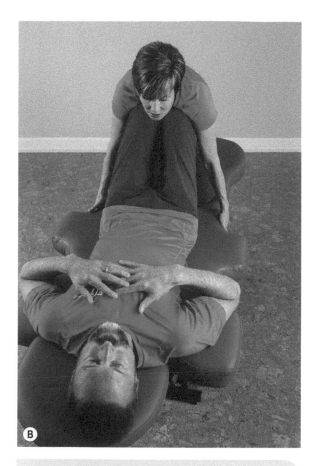

Figure 5.27b
Optional position

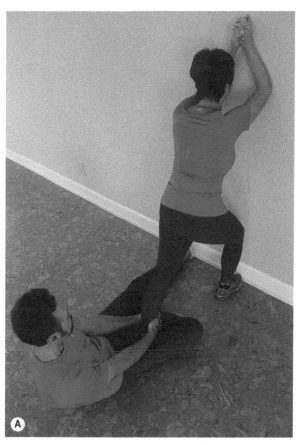

Figure 5.28a
Client leans against wall in lunge position

H. Lunge: Back, Hip, Knee Extension, Ankle Dorsiflexion – Gastrocsoleus – SBN Lower Leg

This should not be painful.

Goal: Target tissues lying within the SBN: soleus and gastrocnemius

Client position: Stands up and leans against the wall in a lunge position.

The client bends both knees and keeps the back heel down on the floor.

Once the practitioner is in position, the client slowly shifts from side to side and then rotates their hips back and forth.

Practitioner:

- Sit behind the client on the floor and cross your legs around the ankle of their back leg. Use your adductors to stabilize the leg.
- Grasp the front of their ankle by interlacing your fingers or stacking hands on top of each other above the ankle bones.

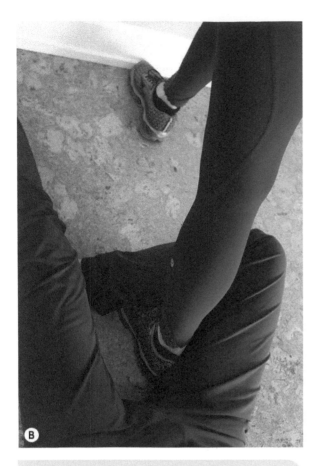

Figure 5.28b
Practitioner leg position

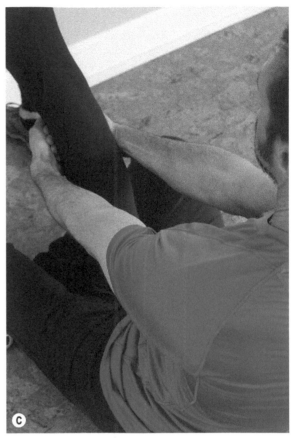

Figure 5.28c
Practitioner leans back

- Think of pulling their tibia behind their femur.
- Slowly move your hands up the front of the client's shin as they continue to press their hips forward.

ROM: Lean your body back.

Traction: Lean back with your entire body as they press their hips forward into the wall.

PNF: "Pull your hips to the wall."

"With your hips still pulling to wall bend your back knee."

"Shift your hips from side to side."

"Rotate your hips around your femur."

Stretch: Move from side to side to increase the stretch while maintaining the traction pulling back on the lower leg.

Repeat: For soleus.

Similar series with straight knee for gastrocs, but bend front knee to target the soleus.

Client positions: Have client move their back foot in closer to the wall.

Repeat: The entire series on the other leg.

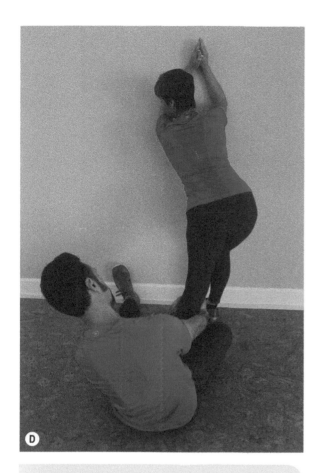

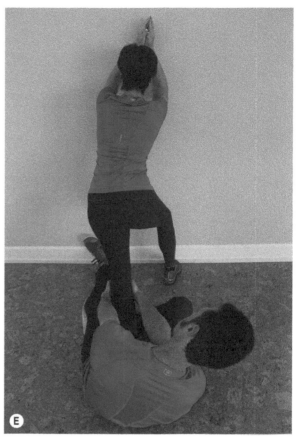

Figure 5.28d
Client shifts hips to right

Figure 5.28e
Client shifts hips to left

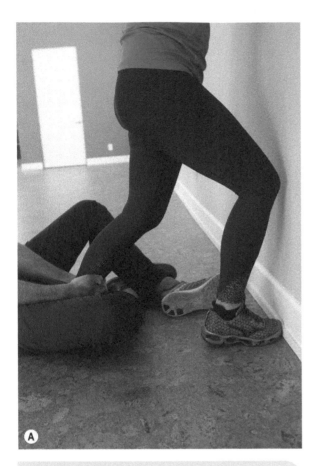

Figure 5.29a
Client bends knee

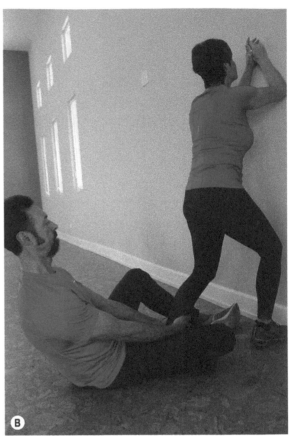

Figure 5.29b
Practitioner leans back for stretch

FST – Upper Body Technique

A. General Evaluation

Supine observations

Before beginning the evaluation, test the client's arm length. Have them actively extend both their arms out at 90° flexion and place their palms together. Then have them continue to flex over their head with palms together, ending as close to 180° as possible without pain. Arms return back to neutral.

1. Make sure the person lying on the table is lined up evenly.
2. Check for overall symmetry. Squat down to get a better look.
3. Check the level and symmetry of their shoulders.
4. Head, ribcage, and pelvis relationship.
5. Check for bony landmarks.
6. Check to see if there is a rounding forward of the shoulders.
7. Shoulder anterior to posterior spring – what is the feel of the tissue?
8. Check for arm length and fingertip length.

The duration of the evaluation changes based on time availability, e.g. a 15 second evaluation for a 15 minute FST session.

B. Side Lying

Shoulder warm-up and assessment

Goal: Scapula ROM warm-up and assessment movement in shoulder girdle.

Client position: Lies on their side with shoulders and knees stacked (pillow in between if needed). Make sure their head is in a neutral position.

Practitioner:

- Practitioner sits on the side of the table behind client.
- Cup your hands over the top of your client's shoulder, with one hand placed over the other.
- Rest their wrist comfortably on your arm.

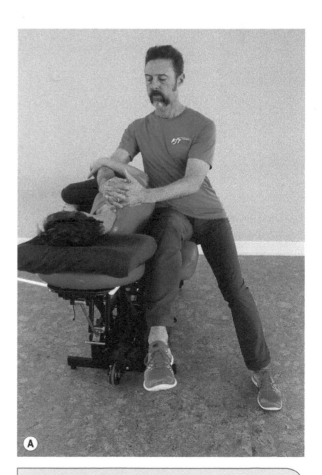

Ⓐ

Figure 6.1a
Practitioner body position

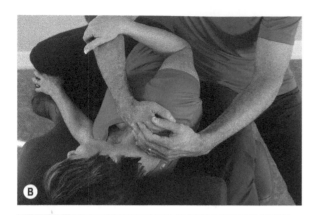

Figure 6.1b
Practitioner hand position

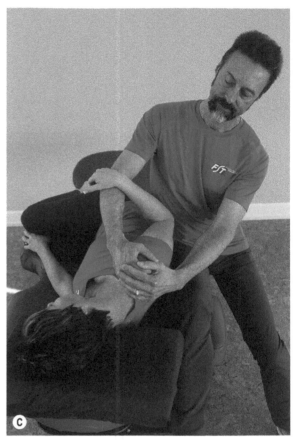

Figure 6.1c
Circumduction

Practitioner:

- Lean forward with your body to begin gently moving the client's shoulder around to check ROM.

- As you circumduct the client's shoulder, allow it to move forward and then downward on the exhalation.

Goal: Target SFAN, DFAN.

Increase retraction.

Client position: Client lies on their side with shoulders and knees stacked. Make sure their head is in a neutral position.

Practitioner:

- With your hand and body in the same position, circle to open their shoulder back into retraction.

- Lean your body weight back into the stretch.

ROM: Open shoulder back into retraction.

Traction: Open shoulder back into retraction.

PNF: Client contracts and pulls their shoulder forward into your hands into protraction.

Cue for PNF: "Pull your shoulder forward into my hands."

Stretch: Increase shoulder retraction.

Repeat: Two or more times.

Goal: Target SFAN and DFAN.

Increase shoulder depression.

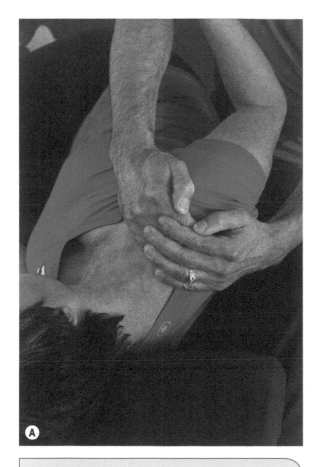

Figure 6.2a
Retraction

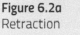

Figure 6.2b
Protraction

Client position: Lies on their side with shoulders and knees stacked.

Practitioner: Traction client's shoulder downward for the stretch.

ROM: Shoulder depression.

Traction: Depress shoulder downward toward top hip.

PNF: Client contracts to elevate shoulder upward in elevation.

Cue for PNF: "Shrug up into my hands."

Stretch: Increase shoulder depression.

Repeat: Two or more times.

Circumduct again. Are there any improvements?

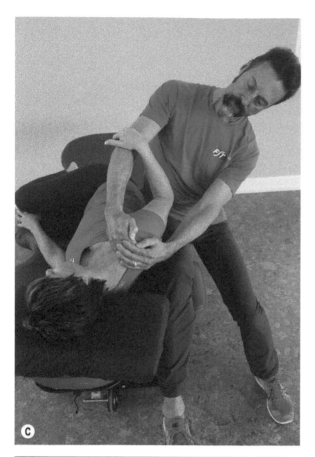

Figure 6.2c
Depression

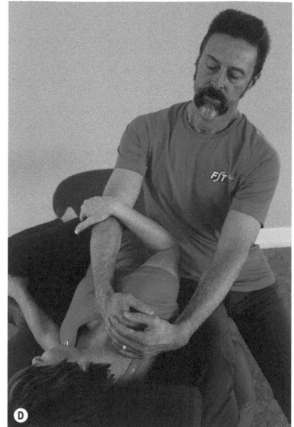

Figure 6.2d
Elevation

C. Range of Motion Evaluation, Warm-up, and FST PNF Stretch

Traction, oscillate and circumduct (TOC) the shoulder and arm anytime within this sequence to ensure the client remains relaxed and the nervous system remains in parasympathetic mode.

1. Traction arm up

Goal: Target tissues within the DBAN: posterior aspect of the shoulder joint. Check for anterior posterior joint glide and restrictions.

Client position: Client lying supine on the table.

Practitioner:

- Grasp client's arm on the lower arm bones to traction their arm upward, keeping their elbow straight. Hands are placed with one hand supporting inside of the client's wrist and other hand supporting at the elbow.

- Traction of the shoulder up at 90° flexion. Rise up into the balls of your feet, keeping your arms relaxed and allowing your body into the movement.

- Stand very close to client and lean slightly over them to have the best leverage. Their arm should be in the center of your body.

- Check for posterior joint glide and restrictions by gently lifting the arm upward.

Traction: Shoulder up at 90° flexion.

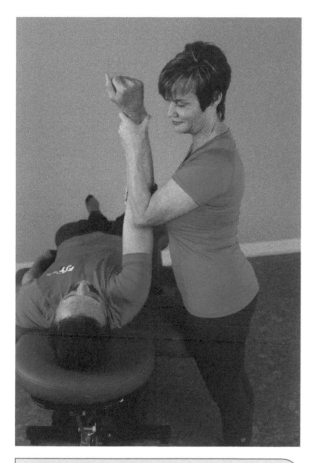

Figure 6.3
Traction arm up

2. Oscillation-circumduction

Goal: To relax the nervous system and give the practitioner an opportunity to begin general assessment of the client's shoulder movement and nervous system.

Client position: Lying supine.

Practitioner:

- Continue on from the previous position, with your hand around the medial aspect of the client's elbow. Your other hand remains on the medial side of their wrist.

- Spend a few moments alternating between traction, oscillation, and circumduction of the shoulder joint in clockwise and counterclockwise directions.

Traction: Shoulder up at 90° flexion.

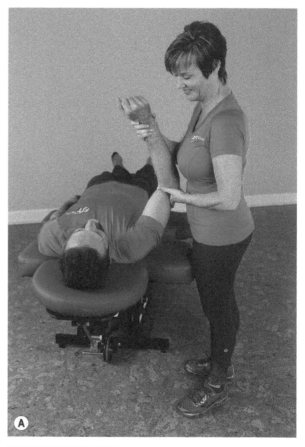

Figure 6.4a
Oscillate-Circumduct (TOC)

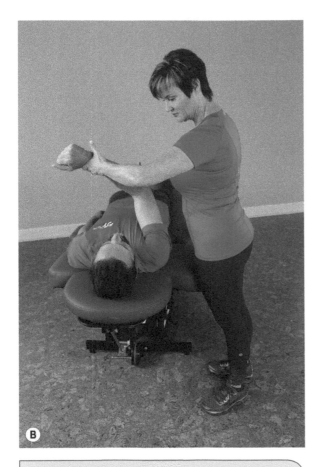

Figure 6.4b
Circumduction

All PNF stretches should be done using traction throughout the stretching process.

3. *Shoulder traction (neutral/loose glenohumeral joint position) – traps, scalenes, joint capsule – SBAN, DBAN*

A. **Goal:** Target tissues within the SBAN, DBAN: upper traps, scalenes, glenohumeral joint capsule.

Client position: Lying supine, reaches out and grasps the practitioner's inside wrist.

Practitioner: Reach up and place outside hand on the front of the client's shoulder.

Practitioner and client hand position: Grasp just above each other's wrists. Step back into a lunge and lean back on the exhalation to traction.

Traction: Depression of shoulder.

B. **Goal:** Target tissues within the SBAN, DBAN: upper traps, scalenes, glenohumeral joint capsule.

Client position: Lying supine, continues to grasp the practitioner's wrist.

Practitioner:

- From the same position, with your outside hand placed around the front of the client's shoulder.

- Remain holding above the client's wrist, while they continue to hold onto yours, for a solid contact.

- Both inhale in the PNF contraction.

- Step back into a lunge and lean your body back on the exhale to traction.

- Gently move their shoulder down into the table and then down toward the foot of the table.

ROM: Depression.

Traction: Shoulder down into deeper depression.

PNF: Client contracts shoulder up in a shrug motion, up toward their ear and into the practitioner's hand.

Cue for PNF: "Shrug up into my hand."

Stretch: Increase shoulder depression.

Repeat: PNF two or more times.

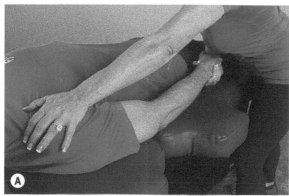

Figure 6.5a
Traction arm down toward foot of table

4. *Shoulder traction (slight flexion/abduction position) – traps, rhomboids, joint capsule – SBAN, DBAN*

Goal: To target tissues within the SBAN: upper traps, rhomboid minor, glenohumeral joint capsule.

Client position: Supine with their arm across your torso.

Practitioner:

- Move the client's arm up to the side, with their hand facing your body and across your torso.

- Hook their hand on your hip for a solid point of contact.

- Place one of your hands above their elbow and the other above their wrist.

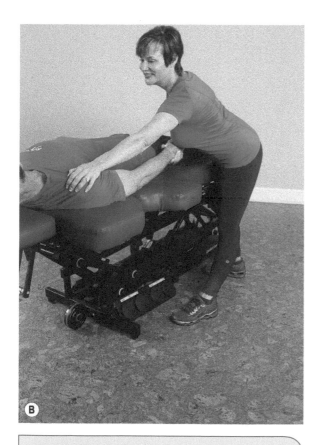

Figure 6.5b
Trap traction down

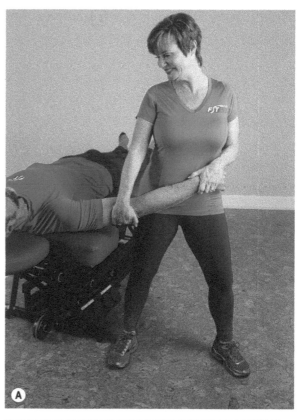

Figure 6.6a
Traction arm out to the side low

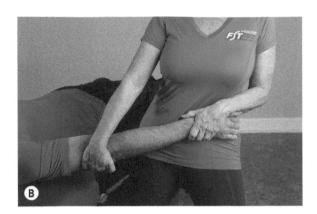

Figure 6.6b
Traction arm out – hand position

ROM: Shoulder depression and arm abduction.

Traction: Arm out to side low-corner pocket of the table.

PNF: Client contracts and shrugs their shoulder and scapula up toward their ear.

Cue for PNF: "Shrug you shoulder toward your ear."

Stretch: Increase shoulder depression and arm abduction.

Repeat: PNF two or more times.

5. Shoulder traction (in 90° abduction) – trap, rhomboids, joint capsule – SFAN, SBAN, DBAN, DFAN, FN

Goal: Target tissues within the SFAN, SBAN, DBAN, DFAN, FN: trap, rhomboids, joint capsule.

To increase shoulder depression and abduction.

Client position: Supine with arm in horizontal flexion.

Practitioner:

- From the previous position, continue to move the client's arm up to the side, with their hand facing your body and across your torso.

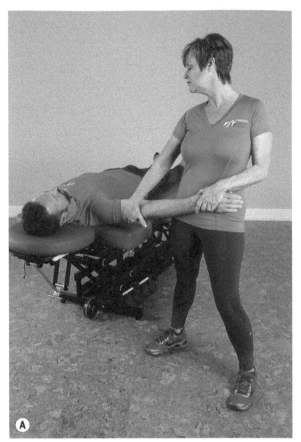

Figure 6.7a
Traction arm out to side at 90° angle

- Hand position remains the same – one of your hands above their elbow and the other above their wrist.

- Use your body to lean away for the ROM and traction.

ROM: Horizontal flexion.

Traction: Slowly increase traction of arm away from their torso.

PNF: Client shrugs their shoulder and scapula up toward their ear.

PNF cue: "Shrug you shoulder toward your ear."

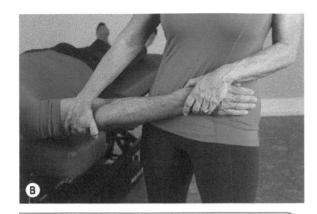

Figure 6.7b
Traction to side close-up

Stretch: Increase shoulder depression and abduction.

Repeat: PNF two or more times.

6. Shoulder traction in transverse, horizontal abduction (at 90°)

– pec major/minor, biceps brachii, coracobrachialis – SFAN, DFAN, FN

Goal: Target tissues within the SFAN, DFAN, FN: anterior chest from the low fibers to high fibers pec major/minor, biceps brachii, coracobrachialis, rotator cuff, joint capsule.

Client position: Supine with their arm out to the side in abduction.

Arm position: Abduction from 45° to 160°.

Practitioner: One hand on client's deltoid-pectoral area. The other hand is above their wrist.

- From the previous position, turn the client's palm to the ceiling.

- Place one hand on their shoulder and the other above their wrist.

- Lower your body to increase the stretch. (Remember to allow your whole body to feel the tissue, not just your hands.)

ROM: Shoulder abduction.

Traction: Arm out and down toward floor on exhale.

PNF: Have client press their entire arm toward the ceiling.

Cue for PNF: "Press your entire arm up to the ceiling."

Stretch: Increase shoulder transverse/horizontal abduction.

Repeat: PNF two or more times.

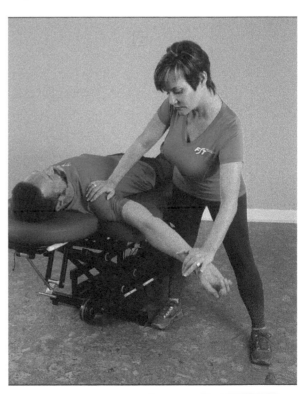

Figure 6.8
Anterior chest – drop arm to floor

7. Shoulder traction (diagonal overhead position) – pec major/minor, coracobrachialis, rhomboids, lats – FN, SFAN, DFAN, DBAN, SBAN

Goal: To target tissues within the FN, SFAN, DFAN, DBAN, SBAN: including pec major/minor, coracobrachialis, rhomboids, lats, rotator cuff. To increase shoulder abduction, flexion.

Client position: Supine with their arm out to the side in abduction and across your torso.

Practitioner:

- One hand holding above their wrist and the other holding above their elbow.

- Lunge away with your body and lean your torso away from table to increase stretch.

ROM: Arm in flexion, moving from 80° to 175°.

Traction: Arm overhead 150° out toward the corner of table on the diagonal.

PNF: Client pulls their scapula down to their opposite hip.

Cue for PNF: "Pull your shoulder blade down toward your opposite hip."

Stretch: Increase shoulder flexion moving from 80° to 175°.

Repeat: PNF two or more times.

Transition: Traction the client's arm up at 90° to clear joint space (see Figure 6.4) before moving their arm to the next position at the top of the table.

Make sure there is no pinching in shoulder. If there is, move their arm into less overhead flexion, more to the corner of the table.

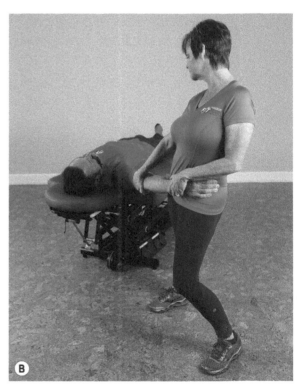

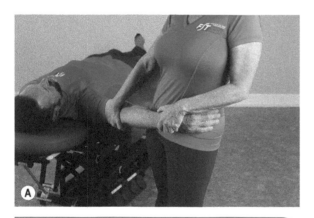

Figure 6.9a
Arm up to diagonal hand position

Figure 6.9b
Traction arm up diagonal

8. Shoulder flexion overhead – pec major/ minor, lat, triceps – FN, SFAN, DFAN, DBAN, SBAN

Overhead shoulder flexion

Goal: To target tissues within the FN, SFAN, DFAN, DBAN, SBAN: pecs, lats, and triceps.

To increase overhead flexion.

Client position: Supine with their arm overhead in shoulder flexion, with arm adducted as comfortably as possible.

Practitioner:

- Lower your body into a squatting position.

- One hand placed above their elbow and your other hand above their wrist.

- Use your body weight to increase the stretch.

ROM: Overhead flexion.

Traction: Traction their arm overhead and continue increasing it after each PNF pass.

PNF:

- Get the client to contract and pull their scapula down toward their feet.

- Get the client to contract and push their arm up toward the ceiling.

Cue for PNF:

- "Pull you shoulder blade down toward your same hip."

- "Lift your arm up to the ceiling."

- Increase traction overhead.

- Move their arm down toward the floor into deeper flexion.

Repeat: Each one or two or more times.

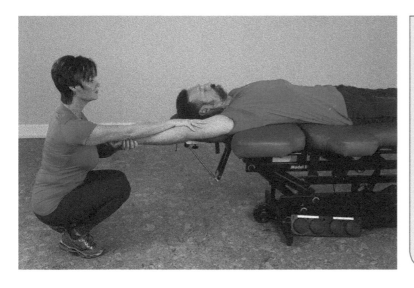

Figure 6.10
Arm overhead to top of table

9. Shoulder flexion overhead with horizontal adduction – rhomboids, lat, triceps – FN, DBAN, SBAN

Transition: Walk the client's arm around into the next position.

(Lift their arm up and over, using repeating StretchWave™ mobilizations before stretching.)

Goal: To target tissues within the FN, DBAN, SBAN: rhomboids, lat, triceps.

To increase overhead flexion and horizontal adduction.

To stretch specific fibers of the lats, rhomboids, functional and back arm nets.

Client position: Lying on side and reaches arm up overhead.

Practitioner:

- Standing at the corner of the table, place one hand on back of client's scapula and other hand on their wrist.
- Client's arm is across your body.
- Lunge and lean away to increase the stretch.

ROM: Overhead flexion and horizontal adduction.

Traction: Arm up overhead into flexion.

PNF: Have them pull their scapula down to their same hip as they roll their body back down to table.

Cue for PNF: "Pull your shoulder blade back down to your same hip and roll your body back down to the table."

Stretch: Increase flexion overhead and horizontal adduction.

Repeat: PNF two or more times.

Transition: Walk their arm down and around toward the bottom corner of the table for the next stretch.

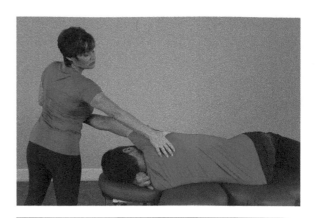

Figure 6.11
Lat – top corner table

10. Shoulder horizontal adduction – traps, deltoid, posterior shoulder joint – SBAN

Goal: To target tissues within the SBAN: – trap, posterior deltoid, and superior posterior shoulder joint.

To increase shoulder depression, adduction.

Client position: Rolls back into a supine position from side lying. Their arm is across their body.

Practitioner:

- From the previous position, remain holding onto the client's wrist and walk down to the end of the table.
- Reach across and place your other hand on their shoulder as you traction their arm across their body.
- Use your body to lean away and increase the stretch.

ROM: Arm in adduction.

Traction: Traction their entire arm across front of body at 45°.

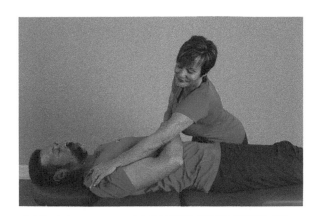

Figure 6.12
Trap across body – low corner pocket

PNF: Have the client pull their arm and shoulder back and away from you and shrug their shoulder.

Cue for PNF: "Shrug up into my hand."

Stretch: Circle shoulder down toward table and around, then increase traction across their body.

Repeat: Two or more times.

Now, to finish the SFAN by moving down to the hands. So often the hands are overworked and underappreciated!

 11. "Dance of the Carpals": hand/ wrist mobilization – carpal joint glides/capsule and tunnel stretch – SFAN, SBAN

Goal: To gently stretch and slowly open up and release the joints and fascial tissue of the hand (carpals, metacarpals, phalanges) by doing the Dance of the Carpals, ending with traction of each finger! And that is what we call giving them some "finger love."

Client position: Supine, with arm across their body.

Practitioner:

- From the previous position, stand up and lean away, focusing on the client's hand.

- Move from the wrist to the last joint of their fingers.

- Using both hands, work from the center of their palm, moving outward to the sides of their hand to open it up. For the fingers, use one hand to stabilize and the other to traction the fingers and thumb.

Traction: Open all carpal, metacarpal, and phalangeal joints and surrounding tissues for wrist, hand, and fingers.

PNF: None.

Cue for PNF: None.

Stretch: This is done with the slow traction and oscillating of each joint of the fingers and thumb.

Repeat if necessary.

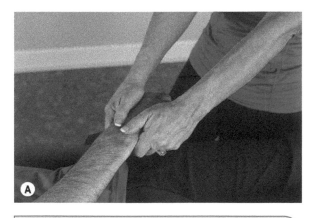

Ⓐ

Figure 6.13a
Dance of the Carpals – hand traction

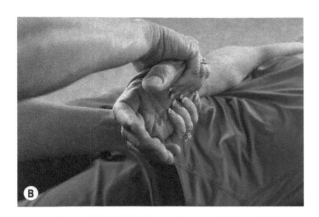

Figure 6.13b
Hand position

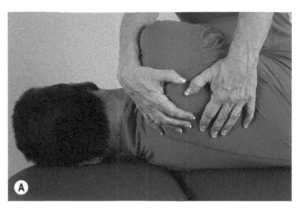

Figure 6.14a
Sweet Roll at shoulder and upper spine

12a. "Sweet Roll": Shoulder protraction, trunk rotation – posterior shoulder and upper back – SN, SBAN, DBAN

This is a signature stretch that is worth spending extra time on.

Goal: To target tissues within the SBAN, DBAN: posterior shoulder and upper back.

To increase upper spinal rotation.

Client position: Supine with their arm across their torso.

Practitioner:

- Place one hand on back of their shoulder and the other on the back of their ribcage.

- Lean your own body into them for a strong contact.

ROM: Spinal rotation.

Traction: Think of lifting the shoulder girdle and ribcage up toward the ceiling and increase rotation.

PNF: Have the client roll their shoulder back down into the table.

Cue for PNF: "Roll your shoulder back down to the table."

Stretch: Increase the spinal rotation.

Repeat: Two or more times.

12b. "Sweet Roll": Full spinal rotation – erector spinae, quadratus lumborum, rhomboids – SN, FN

Goal: To target tissues within the SN, FN: posterior shoulder and back including erector spinae, quadratus lumborum, rhomboids.

To increase spinal rotation.

Client position: Supine with arm across torso.

Practitioner:

- Position one hand on their shoulder and your other hand moves down to their hip on the same side.

- Rotate their torso down toward the table as you press their hip open and back to table.

- Continue moving your top hand down their spine until you have reached their hip as you repeat the PNF.

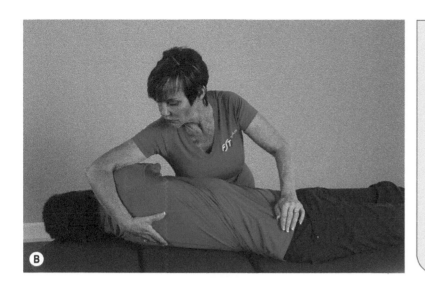

Figure 6.14b
Sweet Roll at shoulder and hip

- Do one last Sweet Roll squeeze of the tissue on the client's exhalation.

ROM: Spinal rotation.

Traction: Think of lifting the shoulder girdle and ribcage up toward the ceiling and increase rotation with your top hand and press their hip back down into the table with your bottom hand.

PNF: Have client roll their entire body back down into the table.

Cue for PNF: "Roll your entire body back down to the table."

Stretch: Increase the spinal rotation in opposite directions for the upper and lower body.

Repeat: Two or more times.

Transition: Continue to walk slowly around the top of the table.

Ask the client to slide over to the side of the table for the next stretch.

13. External rotation – internal rotators – SFAN, DFAN

TIP

Think of the simple cues: traction (out), drop (your body down), lift (hips up). Traction is the key to success for this series.

Goal: To target tissues within the SFAN, DFAN: internal rotators of the cuff. To increase external rotation.

Client position: Supine with their arm out and bent at a 90° angle. Have them move to the edge of the table. They need to be far over enough for the joint to align with the edge of the table. This is necessary so their scapula remains on the table for stability and the humerus can be abducted down toward the floor.

Practitioner:

- Face your body into the table and traction their arm straight up at 90° to begin.

- From the last position, turn so you are facing the top of the table.

- Hook your inside arm around the bend of their elbow and grasp your other arm for stability.

- Place your other hand very gently around the medial aspect of their wrist. Please note this is only a light contact point and should not have any real pressure applied.

- Step away from the table into a parallel lunge, keeping your body squared off.

- Lean away with your hips for the traction.

- Bend at the waist and drop your own body down to achieve the arm abduction.

- Lift your hips up in order to rotate their entire shoulder and arm into deeper external rotation. Do not push down on the arm.

Repeat the sequence for each PNF pass: Out, down, lift.

ROM: External rotation.

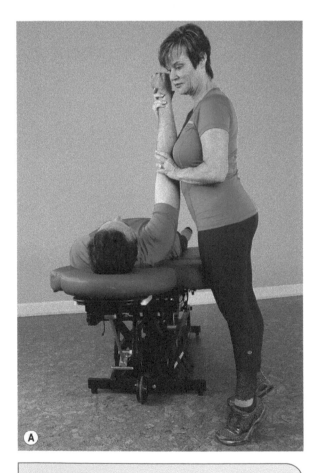

Figure 6.15a
Traction arm up at 90° for preparation

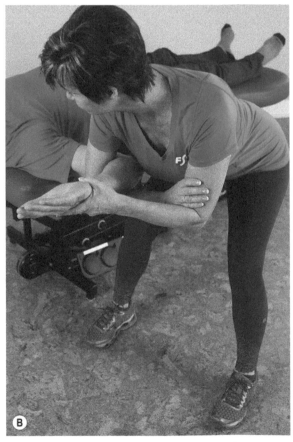

Figure 6.15b
Rotator cuff – external rotation to stretch internal rotators

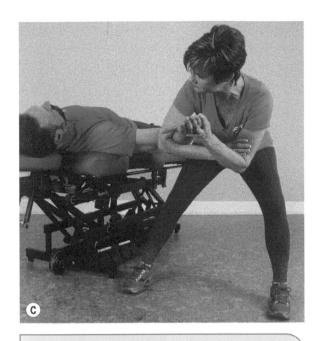

Figure 6.15c
Traction out

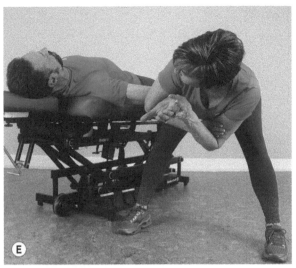

Figure 6.15e
Tilt

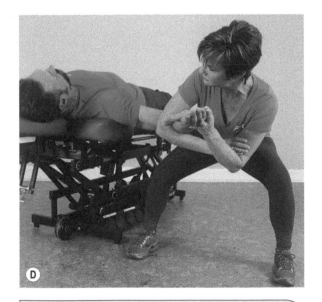

Figure 6.15d
Sink

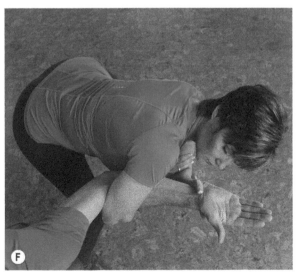

Figure 6.15f
Top view - external

Traction:

- Traction arm up at 90° to begin.

- Traction shoulder out to side at a 90° angle for the shoulder and the elbow.

- Rotate into deeper external rotation by lifting their elbow upward.

PNF: Get the client to internally rotate their entire shoulder toward the ceiling. Traction as you gently stretch it into external rotation.

Cue for PNF: "Press your arm up into me."

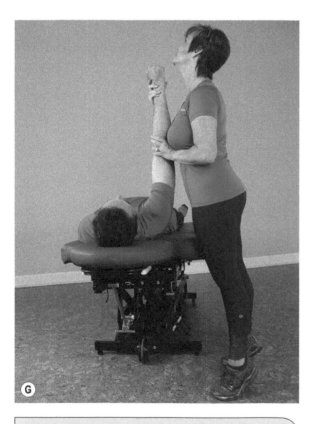

G

Figure 6.15g
Traction arm up at 90°

Stretch: Increase external rotation.

Repeat: Two or more times.

14. Internal rotation – external rotators – DBAN

Goal: To target tissues within the DBAN: internal rotators of the cuff. To increase internal rotation.

Client position: Supine with their arm out to their side and bent at a 70° angle. Get the client to move to the edge of the table – far enough for the joint to align with the edge of the table. This is necessary to allow their scapula to remain on the table for stability.

Practitioner:

- From the last position, turn your body around and face toward the foot of the table.

- Bring the client's arm down to a 70° angle, like putting their hand into their side pocket.

- Align your hips to be at the same angle as their humerus.

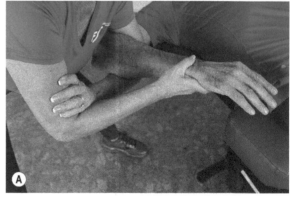

A

Figure 6.16a
Internal rotation to stretch external rotators

- Hook your inside arm around the bend of their elbow and grasp your other arm for stability.

- Place your other hand very gently around the lateral aspect of their wrist. Please note this is only a light contact point and should not have any real pressure applied.

- Step away from the table into a parallel lunge, keeping your body squared off.

- Lean away with your hips for the traction.

- Bend at the waist and drop your body down to achieve the arm abduction.

- Lift your hips up to rotate their entire shoulder and arm into deeper internal rotation. Do not push down on the arm.

Repeat the sequence for each PNF pass: Out, down, lift.

ROM: Internal rotation.

Traction: Traction shoulder out at 70° angle for the shoulder and the elbow. Rotate into deeper internal rotation by lifting their elbow upward.

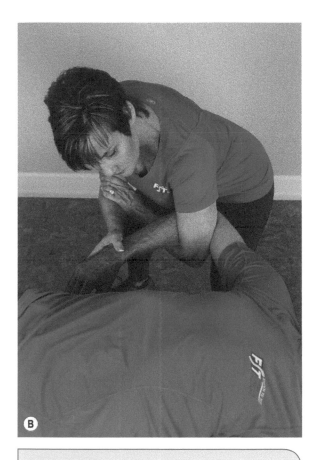

Figure 6.16b
Top view starting position

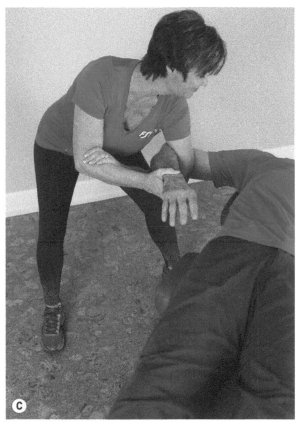

Figure 6.16c
Lean

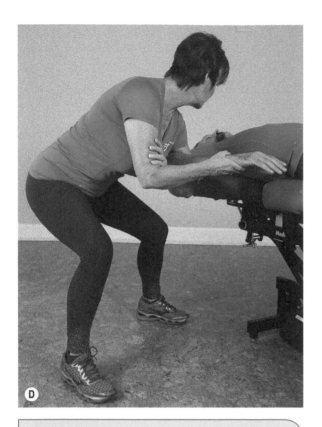

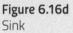

Figure 6.16d
Sink

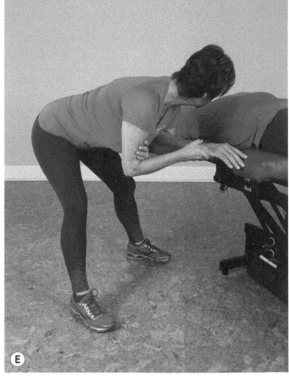

Figure 6.16e
Tilt

PNF: Get the client to externally rotate their entire shoulder toward the floor. Traction as you gently stretch it into internal rotation.

Cue for PNF: "Press your arm up into me."

Stretch: Increase internal rotation.

Repeat: Two or more times.

Repeat the sequence again for each PNF pass: Out, down, lift.

- Face the table and traction the arm up at 90° one more time.

- Turn back around to face the top of the table for the next stretch.

15. Shoulder horizontal abduction/ER (at 90°) – pec major – SFAN, FN

Goal: To target tissues within the SFAN, FN: pec major.

To increase shoulder abduction, external rotation, and elbow extension.

Client position:

- Supine at the edge of the table with their elbow and lower arm completely off the table. They need to be over far enough for the joint to align with the edge of the table. This is necessary to allow their scapula to remain on the table for stability arm at the edge of the table.

- Externally rotate their arm at 90° from the shoulder and elbow.

- Slowly move forearm into full extension at elbow.

Practitioner:

- From the last position, now face the top of the table again, place your inside hand on the outer aspect of their pec major and press it down into the table, with your outside arm.

- Place your outside hand on their distal humerus and wrap your fingers around the medial aspect of the joint.

- Lunge forward onto your inside leg and provide a support for their arm with your leg – like an extension of the table.

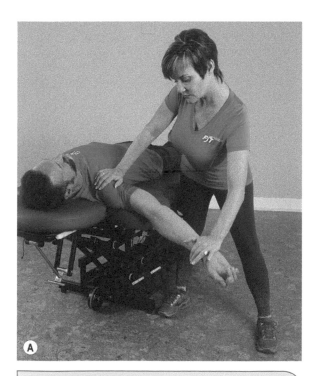

Figure 6.17a
Pec straight arm

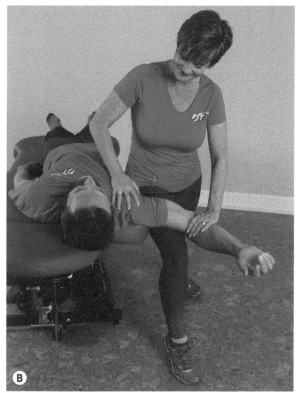

Figure 6.17b
Pec bent arm hand placement

- Use your body instead to increase the stretch by leaning away from the table.

Transitional hand position:

- Move your inside hand down to the medial aspect of their elbow and your outside hand down to the lateral aspect of lower arm bones.

- Finish the stretch by lengthening their elbow joint into full extension.

- Extend your leg supporting their arm to assist in increasing the stretch.

- Shift your weight over your front foot and increase your torso leaning forward at the hips to get a full stretch.

ROM: shoulder abduction, external rotation, and elbow extension.

Traction: Shoulder out at 90°, abduct, externally rotate, and into elbow extension.

PNF:

- Get the client to press their entire arm (maintain a 90° angle) toward their chest by contracting their pecs.

- Contract their arm into internal rotation.

- Have the client do a combination of both movements together by contacting their pecs and rotator cuff.

- Get the client to contract and lift their entire arm up toward the ceiling.

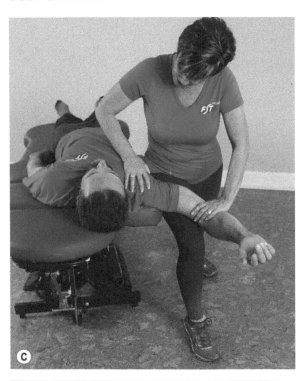

Figure 6.17c
Pec stretch

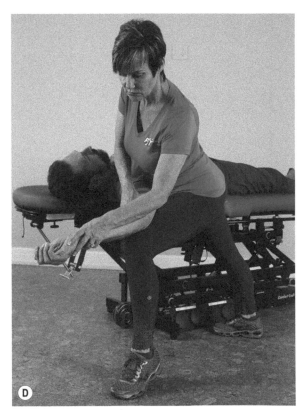

Figure 6.17d
Sternal fibers

Cues for PNF:

- "Press your entire arm up into me" or "Do a pec deck move."

- "Rotate your arm up into me."

- "Now do both press up and rotate."

- "Press your entire arm up to me."

Stretch: Increase external rotation, abduction, and elbow extension.

Repeat: Two or more times.

Finish the stretch by straightening their arm all the way out by extending the elbow and moving their arm down toward the floor to get all fiber angles! Remember to use your body weight, not just your arms.

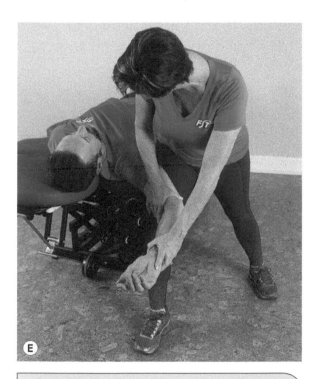

Ⓔ

Figure 6.17e
Final position

16. Setting the shoulder

Just as we did with the sacrum, we feel it is important to stabilize the shoulder girdle after stretching.

- Traction arm up at 90°.

- Traction arm down at neutral.

- Press shoulder and wrist down into table at the same time.

- Place one hand on the front of their shoulder and the other on top of the wrist with their hand flat on the table, palm side down.

- To complete the lengthening, gently pull their fingertips down toward the foot of the table and flatten the palm down into table.

- Gently rocking the entire arm back and forth between the shoulder and wrist, find a still point and pause for a moment ... with your heart over their heart ... and breathe together.

D. ROM Evaluation Warm-up and FST PNF Stretch

Key points that are especially important for neck work:

1. There is a much higher level of sensitivity in the neck area due to the extensive amount of neural and other delicate and/or sensitive tissue.

2. It is often the most protected and personal area on someone and needs to be handled with the utmost care.

3. It is the ultimate area to work as far as trust is concerned.

4. There is an even stronger need for the client to feel confidence from the practitioner.

5. Slow, gentle movements are important.

6. Work seated, if possible, so you can have minimal tension in your own body.

7. Move through another pathway following the stretch to return back to neutral.

8. Remember: less is more – especially with neck work!

Neck work: Do stretches 4–7 to one side then repeat on the other side.

1. Shoulder depression – bilateral traps – SBAN

Goal: To target tissues within the SBAN: traps.

To settle the shoulders down and bring client to a more parasympathetic state.

Client position: Supine and relaxed.

Practitioner:

- Place both of your hands on the top of client's shoulders with your fingertips lifted.

- Press their shoulder down toward their feet.

- "Kitty Cat" move by alternately pressing one shoulder down at a time.

ROM: Depression of shoulders.

Traction: None.

PNF: Have them shrug into your hands.

Cue for PNF: "Shrug up into my hands."

Stretch: Increase shoulder depression.

Repeat: PNF two or more times.

2. Neck traction – cranial/cervical joint capsules and tissues – SBAN, DBAN, SBN, DFN

Client position: Supine and relaxed.

Goal: To target tissues within the SBAN, DBAN, SBN, DFN: suboccipitals, decompress upper cervical joints and increase relaxation through parasympathetic activation.

Practitioner: Preferably seated (note that there are many ways to do this).

- Place your hands on the back of their neck down toward C7 to begin and put fingertips into the laminar grove on either side of the spine.

- Slowly move along the tissue one vertebra at a time until your hands land under the client's occipital ridge.

- Allow your hands to gently sink into the tissue at each section as you traction up toward their head.

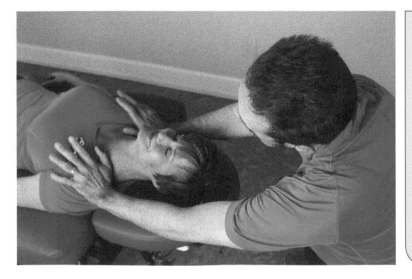

Figure 6.18
Shoulder depression

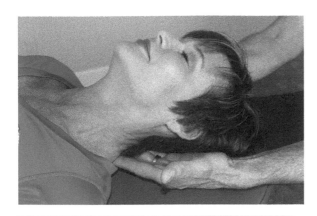

Figure 6.19
Neck traction

- Lean back in your chair to increase the stretch by using your body – not just your hands.

ROM: Cranial/upper cervical decompression.

Traction: Gently press in toward the center of the neck, as you simultaneously traction by hooking the mastoids and lean back to finish this move.

PNF: None.

Cue for PNF: None.

Stretch: Increase space between the cranium and atlas, and on through the upper cervical joints while stretching all tissues overlying the same and on down through the neck as far as possible.

Repeat: Two or more times.

3. Suboccipital traction ROM – subcranial joint capsule, tissues – SBN, SBAN, DBAN

Goal: To target tissues within the SBN, SBAN, DBAN: decompress cranial cervical and upper cervical joints, stretch cervical joint capsules and all overlying tissues, stimulate parasympathetic state, increase relaxation.

Client position: Supine and relaxed.

Practitioner: From last position:

- Slowly slide along the tissue until your hands land under the client's occipital ridge.

- Allow your fingertips to gently palpate as you lengthen their SBN.

- Curl your finger pads up and around their occipital ridge.

- Allow the weight of their head to really drop into your hands.

- Use a mini StretchWave™ motion.

ROM: Upper cervical traction, flexion.

Traction: Lean back in your chair to increase the traction and stretch of upper cervical joints using your body and not just your hands.

PNF: None.

Cue for PNF: None.

Stretch: Increase upper cervical flexion, decompress upper cervical joints.

Repeat: Two or more times.

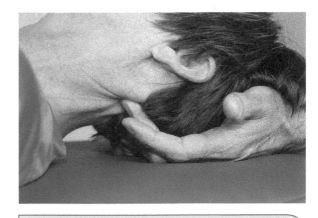

Figure 6.20
Suboccipital neck traction, ROM

4. Traction, upper cervical flexion – cervical/upper thoracic extensors – SBN, SBAN, DBAN

Goal: To target tissues within the SBN: extensors of the neck and upper back.

Client position: Supine and relaxed.

Practitioner:

- Place both of your hands on their occipital ridge – cup their head.

- Turn your fingertips slightly so they are now pointed up to the ceiling.

- The heels of your hands are under the occiput for a firm contact.

- Lift their head upward toward the ceiling with traction.

- Increase the stretch by maintaining traction as you guide their chin to their chest into gentle flexion.

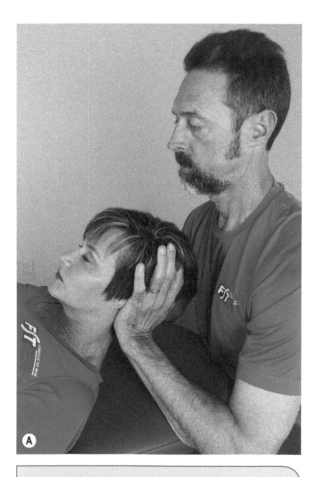

A

Figure 6.21a
Traction in flexion

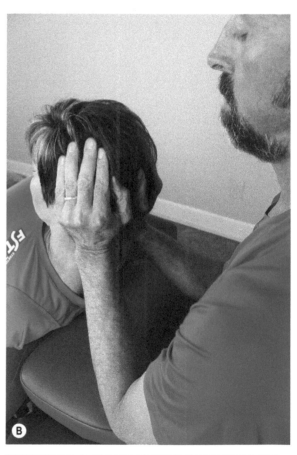

B

Figure 6.21b
Hand position

- Be careful not to restrict their airway.

- Use care when releasing the stretch back to starting position by supporting their head, moving slowly.

- Encourage the cervical curve as their heads floats back down.

- Repeat points 2–6 again for best results.

ROM: Neck flexion.

Traction: Gently traction head up toward ceiling and into flexion.

PNF: Get the client to gently push their head back into your hands in extension.

Cue for PNF: "Gently push your head back into my hands."

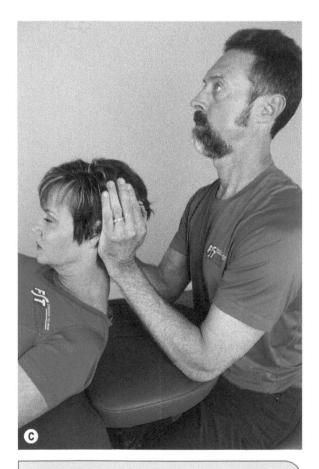

Figure 6.21c
Full flexion

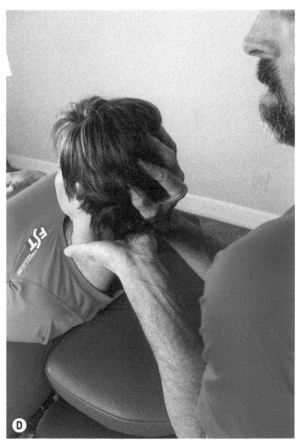

Figure 6.21d
Release

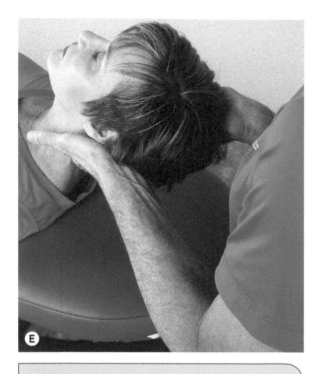

Figure 6.21e
Float down

Stretch: Increase neck flexion.

Repeat: PNF two or more times. Mobilize varied angles to find then stretch all of the tight fibers.

5. Neck rotation right – left cervical rotators – LN, SN, FN

Goal: To target tissues within the LN, SN, FN: cervical rotators (in this case, left side)

To increase neck rotation to the right.

Client position: Supine with head rotated to the right, but slightly less than their full ROM. Once the shoulder is fully depressed down, then the range that remains can be found by turning the head into deeper rotation. As always, only moving as far as is comfortable. Make sure their head is only in rotation and not in any forward or lateral flexion or extension.

Practitioner:

- Repeat traction to begin top of the shoulder.

- Place one hand on the top of their shoulder and use your own shoulder to visualize gliding

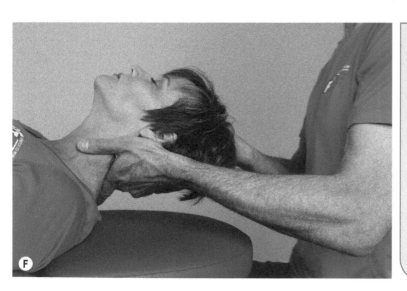

Figure 6.21f
Traction in neutral

the scapula down their ribcage to stabilize their shoulder down into starting position.

- Other hand is placed around the back of the head to move them into rotation.

- Be careful to avoid their eyes by keeping your elbow lifted out to the side.

- Turn the client's head to the right side on the table.

- Use your body to lean to the side to increase the stretch.

- Upon release of PNF, slowly increase ROM of rotation, while maintaining the shoulder depression.

- Slowly circle their head around through flexion and float it back into extension to return to neutral to finish.

ROM: Neck rotation.

Traction: Think of creating space between their shoulder and neck.

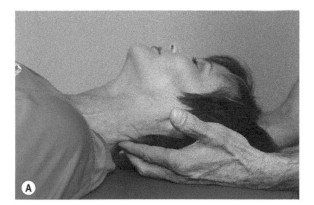

Figure 6.22a
Traction

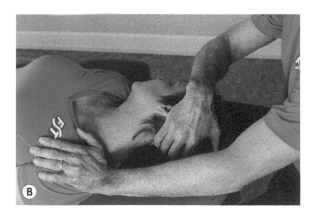

Figure 6.22b
Hand position

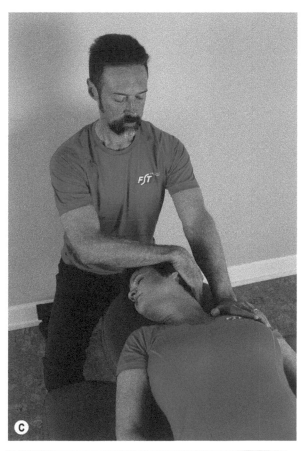

Figure 6.22c
Beginning position

PNF: Client turns eyes and head to opposite direction.

Cue for PNF: "Turn your eyes and head to the ceiling."

Stretch: Increase neck rotation to the right.

Repeat: PNF two or more times. Play with angles to find all of the tight fibers.

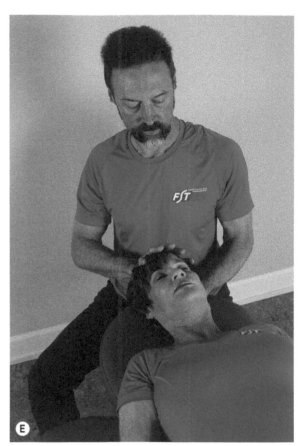

Figure 6.22e
Return to neutral

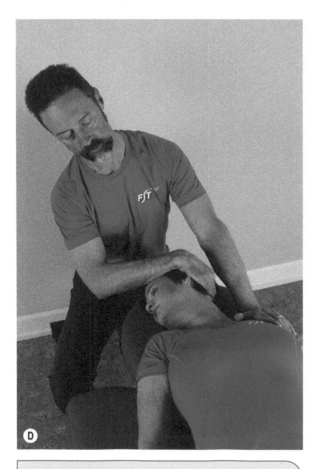

Figure 6.22d
Lean to side

6. Neck lateral flexion right – left lateral flexors – LN, SN, SBN, SBAN, DBAN, DFN

Goal: To target tissues within the LN, SN, SBN, SBAN, DBAN, DFN: lateral fibers of the neck (in this case, left side).

To increase lateral flexion.

Client position: Supine with neck side bent into lateral flexion.

Practitioner:

- Keep the back of the client's head on the table, slide it to the right, moving the ear toward their shoulder.

- Place both of your hands around the base of their neck and move their head into lateral flexion to find their R1 to begin.

- Bring their back into slightly less lateral flexion before gliding the scapula down into slight depression.

- Place your outside hand on the top of client's shoulder and the other hand on the base of their neck.

- Gently press down on their outside shoulder moving the scapula down the ribcage into depression to stabilize.

- Then lean back to traction head and then lean away from the center to stretch their head away from their shoulder.

- Keep the pin down on the shoulder to maintain the stretch.

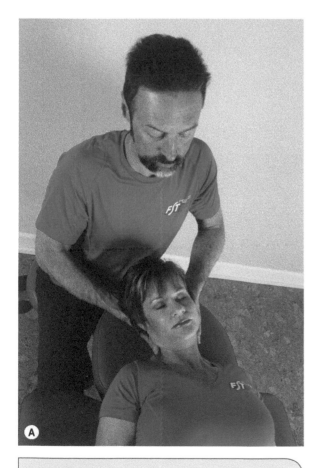

Figure 6.23a
Lateral flexion

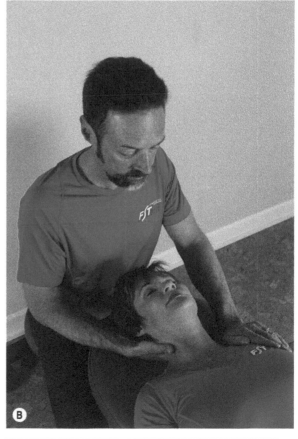

Figure 6.23b
Hand position

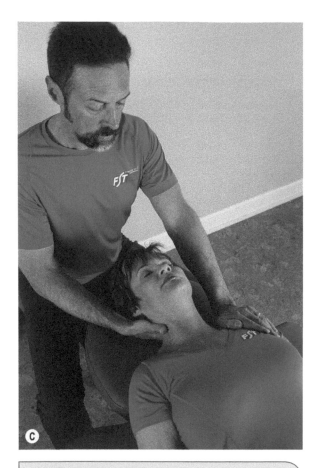

Figure 6.23c
Lean back

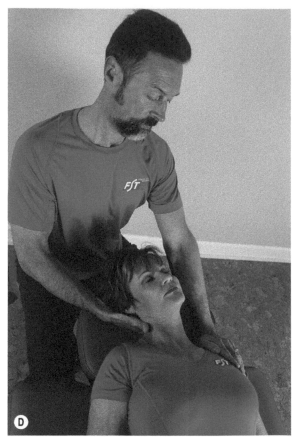

Figure 6.23d
Lean and arc

- Be careful not to let their head tilt backwards and keep their nose pointed to ceiling.

- Increase ROM by gently pressing down on their shoulder as you increase their neck flexion with traction.

- Upon release of PNF, gently and slowly increase shoulder depression and neck flexion.

- Slowly circle their head around through flexion and float it back into extension to return to neutral to finish.

ROM: Lateral flexion.

Traction: Think of creating space between their shoulder and neck.

PNF:

- Have client shrug their left shoulder up into your hand.

- Have the client try to push their head gently back into your hand.

Cue for PNF:

- "Shrug your shoulder up into my hand."

- "Press your head back into my hand."

Stretch: Increase lateral flexion.

Repeat: PNF two or more times. Play with angles to find all of the tight fibers.

Neck traction to finish stretch.

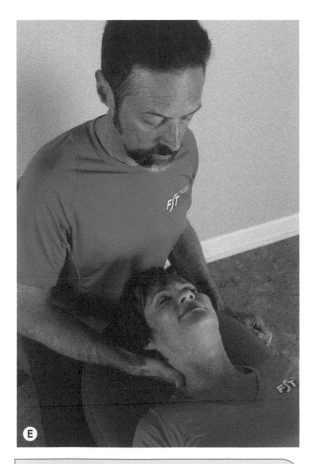

Figure 6.23e
Traction finish

7. Suboccipital traction – subcranial joint capsule, tissues – SBN, SBAN, DBAN

Goal: To target tissues within the SBN, SBAN, DBAN: subcranial joint capsule, tissues.

Client position: Supine and relaxed.

Practitioner:

- Slowly slide along the tissue until your hands land under client's occipital ridge.

- Again allow your fingertips to gently palpate as you lengthen their SBN.

- Curl your finger pads up and around their occipital ridge.

- Allow the weight of their head to really drop into your hands.

- Use mini StretchWave™ motion.

ROM: Upper neck flexion.

Traction: Lean back in your chair to increase the traction and stretch using your body and not just your hands.

PNF: None.

Cue for PNF: None.

Stretch: Increase upper neck flexion.

Repeat: Two or more times.

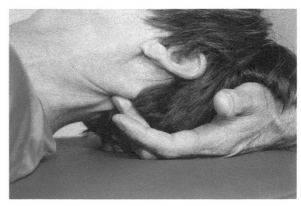

Figure 6.24
Suboccipital traction

8. Traction

- Place your hands on the back of the client's neck down toward C7 to begin and put fingertips into the laminar grove on either side of the spine.

- Slowly move along the tissue one vertebra at a time until your hands land under the client's occipital ridge.

- Allow your hands to gently sink into the tissue at each section as you traction up toward their head.

- Lean back in your chair to increase the stretch by using your body – not just your hands.

ROM: Cranial/upper cervical decompression.

Traction: Gently press in toward the center of the neck, as you simultaneously traction by hooking the mastoids and lean back to finish this move.

PNF: None.

Cue for PNF: None.

Stretch: Increase space between the cranium and atlas, and on through the upper cervical joints, while stretching all tissues overlying the same and on down through the neck as far as possible.

Repeat: Two or more times.

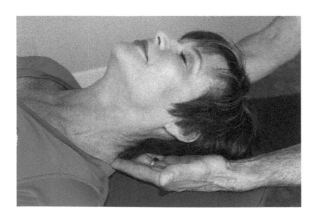

Figure 6.25
Neck traction

9. Full traction – cranial cervical joint capsules, overlying tissues – SBN, SBAN, DBAN

Goal: To target tissues within the SBN, SBAN, DBAN: increase general neck ROM, decompress cranial cervical joints and stretch overlying tissues, increase relaxation.

Client position: Supine and relaxed.

Practitioner: Preferably seated.

- Place one hand below and hook occipital ridge, place other hand outside shoulder; or both hands can be on the base of their neck.

ROM: Traction, decompression.

Traction:

- Hook your hand around base of their neck as you lean body back.

- Progress from light to deeper traction as tolerated.

- Lean back in your chair to increase the stretch using your body and not just your hands.

PNF: None.

Cue for PNF: None.

Stretch: Increase cervical joint space and tissue length.

Repeat: Two or more times.

10. "Crown Set"

Goal: To stabilize and very gently compress the cranium and neck joints.

Allow musculature to stabilize and reset the proprioception.

Client position: Supine.

Practitioner: Seated or kneeling so their hands are in alignment with the top of client's head.

- Place both of your hands together with the heels of hands touching and gently wrapped around the top of their head.

- Apply only a few ounces of pressure for the cranial bones to settle.

- Allow a few breaths together to occur and find a still point.

Practitioner: Standing.

- With the client's head on the table, place your hands one stacked on top of the other on their forehead and apply only a few ounces of pressure.

- Gently tuck client's chin in as they lengthen the back of their neck.

- Hold this position for a few moments as they breathe and relax.

- Find a still point, positioning your heart above their heart, and breathe together.

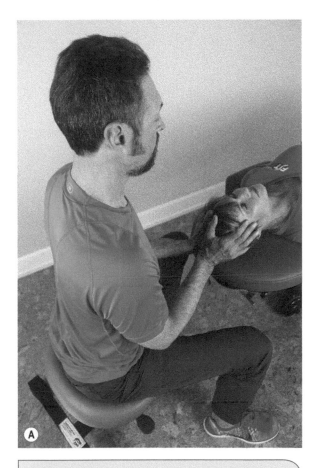

Figure 6.26a
"Crown Set"

11. "Cranium Set": subcranial flexion – craniocervical extensors – DFN

Goal: To stabilize the neck musculature and reset the proprioception.

Client position: Supine.

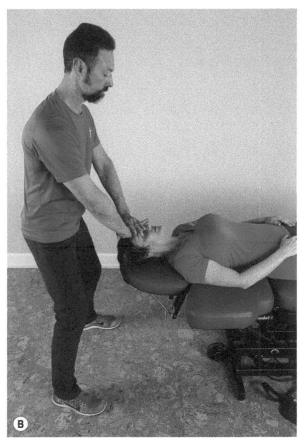

Figure 6.26b
"Cranium Set" full view

12. Shoulder depression – bilateral traps – SBAN – repeat once more to finish

Goal: To target tissues lying within the SBAN: traps.

To settle shoulders down and check to see if there are any changes in the tissue.

Client position: Supine and relaxed.

Practitioner:

- Place both of your hands on the top of the client's shoulders with your fingertips lifted.

- Press their shoulders down toward feet.

- "Kitty Cat" move by alternating pressing one shoulder down at a time.

ROM: Depression of shoulders.

Traction: None.

Stretch: Increase shoulder depression.

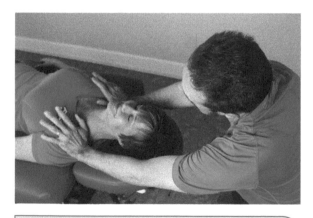

Figure 6.27
Shoulder depression

E. Sitting Stretches

1. Shoulder extension/adduction – anterior deltoid and pecs – SFAN, FN

Goal: To target tissues lying within the SFAN, FN: anterior deltoid and pecs.

To increase extension, shoulder abduction, horizontal abduction, and lateral rotation of the humerus.

Client position: Sitting with their feet hip distance apart and firmly planted flat on the floor. Get them to take their arms behind their body in abduction and interlace their fingers.

Practitioner:

- Wrap your arms around the client above their elbows and gently squeeze them together.

- Grasp your own arms for support, if needed.

- On their exhalation, squeeze their elbows closer together as they lift their chest up.

ROM: Extension, shoulder abduction, horizontal abduction, and lateral rotation of the humerus.

Traction: Think of opening their chest as you pull their elbows closer.

PNF: Get them to contract their chest and anterior shoulders to pull away and out of your hold.

Cue for PNF: "Pull your arms forward and out of my hold."

Stretch: Increase extension, shoulder abduction, horizontal abduction, and lateral rotation of the humerus.

Repeat: PNF two or more times.

2. Shoulder extension/adduction, elbow flexion – anterior deltoid, pecs, anterior joint capsule – SFAN, FN

Goal: To target tissues lying within the SFAN, FN: anterior deltoid, sternal fibers of pecs, anterior glenohumeral joint capsule.

To increase extension, shoulder abduction, horizontal abduction, and lateral rotation of the humerus.

Client position: Sitting with their feet hip distance apart and firmly planted flat on the floor. Get them to take their arms behind their body in abduction and interlace their fingers, while keeping their posture upright.

Practitioner:

- From the last stretch, flatten your palms against the client's back and press into it.

- On their exhalation, lift their arms higher and squeeze their elbows closer together as they lift their chest up.

- Keep walking your hands up their back and maintain their elbows moving closer.

- Use your body to lift their arms up – not just your arms.

ROM: Extension, shoulder abduction, horizontal abduction, and lateral rotation of the humerus.

Traction: Think of pressing their sternum forward as their arms float upwards.

PNF: Get the client try to pull away, out of the hold.

Cue for PNF: "Pull your arms up and out of my hold."

Stretch: Increase extension, shoulder abduction, horizontal abduction, and lateral rotation of the humerus.

Repeat: PNF two or more times. Play with the angles to target more fibers.

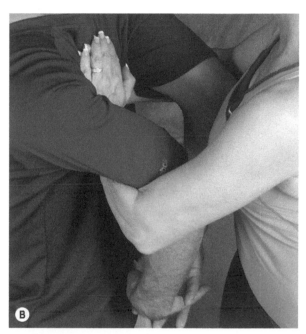

Figure 6.28b
Close up of hand position

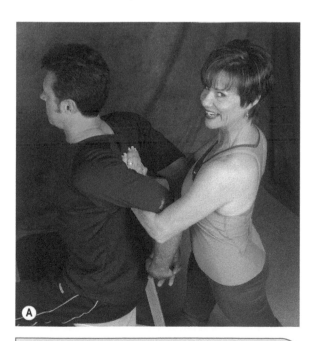

Figure 6.28a
Shoulder extension/adduction, elbow flexion

3. Hands behind head: shoulder abduction, elbow flexion – pec major, anterior chest – SFAN, FN

Goal: To target tissues lying within the SFAN, FN: all the fibers of the anterior chest, pec major.

To increase extension, shoulder abduction, horizontal abduction, and lateral rotation of the humerus.

Client position: Sitting with their feet on the floor, get them to take their arms behind their body in abduction and interlace their fingers. Allow them to arch back a little bit.

Practitioner: Place your hand around and on the outsides of their elbows.

ROM: Increase extension, shoulder abduction, horizontal abduction, and lateral rotation of the humerus.

Traction: Gently traction elbows upward toward ceiling and open back to stretch.

PNF: On PNF have client try to close their elbow toward their face.

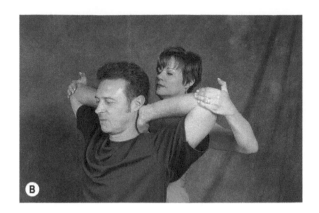

Figure 6.29b
Pec major

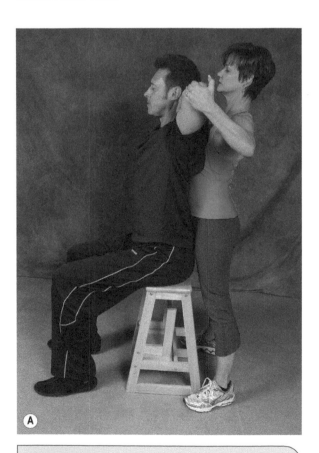

Figure 6.29a
Pec major (anterior chest)

Cue for PNF: "Squeeze your elbows together."

Stretch: Increase extension, shoulder abduction, horizontal abduction and lateral rotation of the humerus.

Repeat: PNF two or more times. Play with the angles to target more fibers.

4. Sitting lats: shoulder abduction, elbow flexion – lats, teres major, QL and intercostals – FN, SN, DFN, LN, DBAN

This stretch targets a great many tissues and hits multiple angles and fibers. So really explore the potential here!

Goal: To target tissues lying within the FN, SN, DFN, LN, and DBAN: lats, teres major, QL, and intercostals.

To increase flexion, lateral rotation, and abduction of humerus, lateral flexion, rotation, and extension of the trunk.

Client position: Sitting with their feet hip distance apart and firmly planted flat on the floor.

- Get the client to lengthen their spine upward.

- Then get them to reach their arm up overhead, then bend elbow behind back into flexion.

Practitioner:

- Stand behind your client with your feet firmly planted, hip distance apart.

- Make sure you are close enough to have contact with the client's back so you can steer them through the stretch.

- As client reaches their arm up into flexion, assist by tractioning arm upward and lift it to clear joint.

- Wrap your arm around the front of their arm and place your hand on the medial side of their elbow. Your other hand grasps the medial aspect of their wrist.

- Continue tractioning up from the elbow.

- On stretch, traction up and over to the side, lifting their arm upward and back into you.

- Use your body to help guide their movement and increase traction.

ROM: Flexion, lateral rotation and abduction of humerus, lateral flexion, rotation and extension of the trunk.

Traction: Think of creating space between the top of the pelvis and the humerus.

PNF: Have client contract and bend laterally to one side. They will attempt to pull their elbows and ribs toward the floor.

Cue for PNF: "Pull your body down toward your hip."

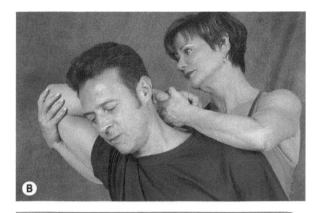

Figure 6.30b
PNF

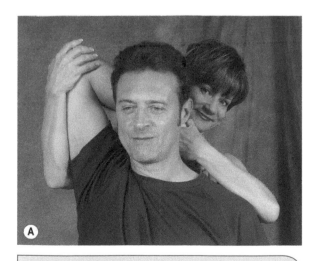

Figure 6.30a
Sitting lats starting position

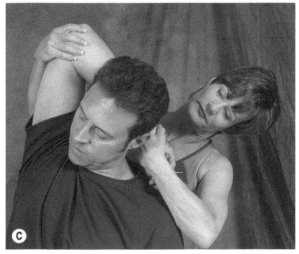

Figure 6.30c
Stretch

Stretch: Increase flexion, lateral rotation and abduction of humerus, lateral flexion, rotation and extension of the trunk

Repeat: PNF two or more times. Play with the angles to target more fibers.

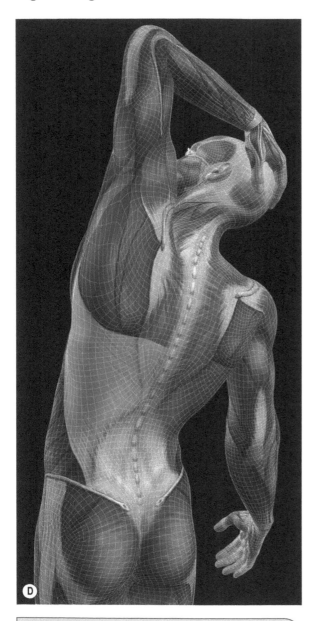

Figure 6.30d
Target tissues within primarily the Functional and Lateral nets

5. Sitting lats: shoulder abduction, elbow flexion, trunk rotation – lats, teres major, QL and intercostals – FN, SN, DFN, LN, and DBAN

Rotation component

Open chest stretch

From the last stretch, to add another component of rotation PNF.

Goal: To target tissues lying within the FN, SN, DFN, LN, and DBAN: lats, teres major, QL, and intercostals.

To target the fibers involved in rotation component.

To increase flexion, lateral rotation and abduction of humerus, lateral flexion, rotation and extension of the trunk.

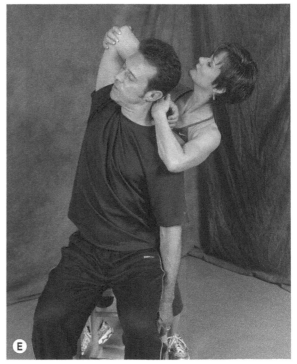

Figure 6.30e
Sitting lats with rotation

Client position: Sitting, as for previous position.

Practitioner: Standing, as for previous position. Lean away with your body to increase traction and stretch.

ROM: Flexion, lateral rotation and abduction of humerus, lateral flexion, rotation, and extension of the trunk.

Traction: Think of creating space between the top of the pelvis and the humerus.

PNF: Get the client to twist torso and pull their elbow down toward the opposite hip.

PNF cue: "Pull you elbow down to your opposite knee."

Stretch: Increase flexion, lateral rotation and abduction of humerus, lateral flexion, rotation and extension of the trunk.

Repeat: PNF series two or more times. Play with the angles to target more fibers.

6. Sitting triceps: shoulder abduction, elbow flexion – triceps – DBAN

Sitting triceps

Goal: To target tissues lying within the DBAN: triceps.

To increase flexion of the elbow, long head of triceps, flexion of the humerus.

Client position: The same as the previous position.

Practitioner: From the last position:

- To focus on the long head of the triceps proximal fibers, change your hands and place the one that was on their elbow in the front of their shoulder and the one that was on their wrist, on their elbow.

- Lift arm upward with gentle traction and assist the client to bend their elbow behind their back.

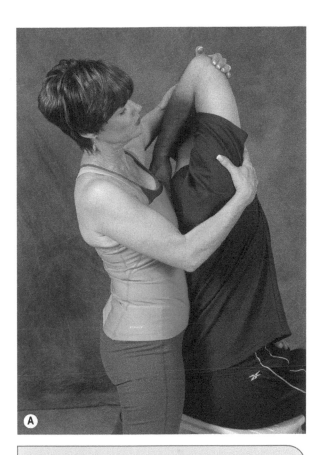

Ⓐ

Figure 6.31a
Sitting triceps PNF (target proximal fibers)

- Then change your hands for the next position with one hand on the back of their elbow and the other on their fingertips.

- While stretching, lift their elbow upward and back into flexion.

- Pull their fingertips down their back.

- While stretching gently pull their hand down their back and press shoulder deeper into extension.

ROM: Flexion of the elbow, long head of triceps flexion of the humerus.

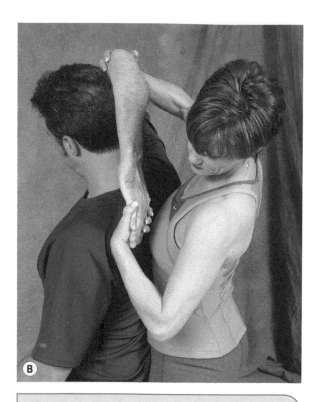

Figure 6.31b
Triceps starting position

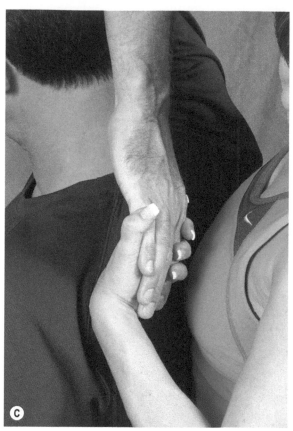

Figure 6.31c
Close up – hand position

Traction: Think of lifting their elbow up toward the ceiling, then back toward you and finally pulling their arm down their back through the fingertips.

PNF: Get the client to push their elbow forward into your hand and try to extend their hand upward.

Cue for PNF: "Push your elbow forward into my hand" and "Try to extend you hand to the ceiling."

Stretch: Increase flexion of the elbow, long head flexion of the humerus. Play with the angles to target more fibers.

Repeat: Two or more times.

7. Levator scapulae release: neck rotation, side flexion same side – levator scapula – DBAN

Neck and shoulder release

Goal: To target tissues lying within the DBAN: levator scapulae. Because this area has been in a contracted state for some time from previous sequences, it is quite nice to release it with this last stretch to finish the sitting series.

Practitioner:

- Release the client's arm from the stretch position from the previous move, in the triceps stretch.

- Assist their head down into forward flexion and around to opposite shoulder.

- Place one hand on their shoulder and the other on the side of the head.

- Gently press downward with both hands.

- Stretch them away from each other.

- Take several breaths to give the tissue time to release.

- Move their head back down through forward flexion and lift it upwards to finish.

- It is important to remember to always move through neutral when returning from a stretch. This is so the tissue that has just been lengthened will not re-contract.

Repeat: 4–6 on the other side.

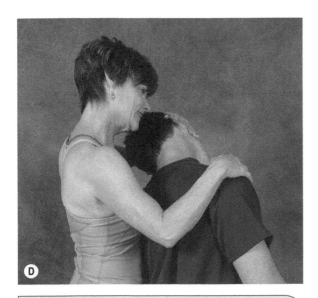

Figure 6.31d
Levator release

F. Floor Stretches

1. Pec major on ball: shoulder abduction, elbow flexion – pec major – SFAN, FN

Goal: To target tissues lying within the SFAN, FN: all the fibers in the anterior chest and shoulder, pec major.

To increase shoulder abduction, horizontal abduction and lateral rotation of the humerus, and back extension.

Client position: Lies supine, arched over a ball with their feet hip distance apart, feet flat on the floor. Fingers are interlaced behind their head.

Practitioner:

- Stand behind the client in a lunge position and lean forward.

- Place your hands on their elbows.

- Gently open their elbows down toward the floor.

- Drop your body down onto your back knee.

- Lean forward to increase the stretch.

- To further increase the stretch and target more pec fibers, slowly roll the ball toward the feet.

ROM: Shoulder abduction, horizontal abduction and lateral rotation of the humerus and back extension.

Traction: Think of opening their shoulders away from their torso and down to the floor.

PNF: Get the client to press their elbows toward the ceiling.

Cue for PNF: "Pull your elbows together."

Stretch: Increase shoulder abduction, horizontal abduction and lateral rotation of the humerus, and back extension.

Repeat: PNF two or more times. Play with the angles to target more fibers.

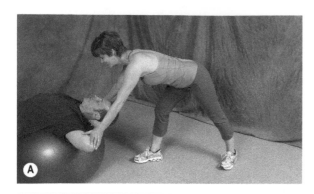

Figure 6.32a
Pec major on ball – starting position

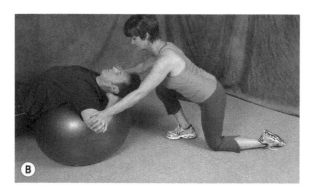

Figure 6.32b
Practitioner kneels down

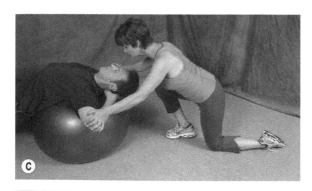

Figure 6.32c
Practitioner leans forward

2. Pec minor on ball: shoulder abduction, elbow flexion (90°/90°) – pec minor – DFAN

Goal: To target tissues lying within the DFAN: all the fibers deep in the chest, pec minor.

To open all three angles and slips of the pec minor. To increase retraction of the scapula.

Client position:

- Kneeling with their knees hip distance apart and one arm placed on a ball, elbow bent at a 90° angle. The ball should be about the same height as they are when on all fours.

- Place their other hand on the floor directly underneath their shoulder.

- Get them to rotate their torso slowly and gently down toward their hand on the floor.

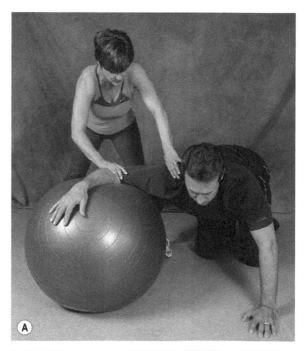

Figure 6.33a
Pec minor on ball – starting position

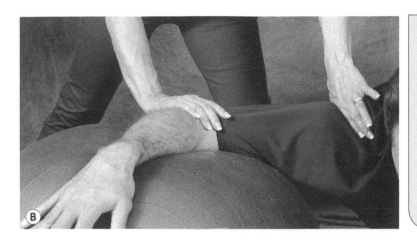

Figure 6.33b
Hand position

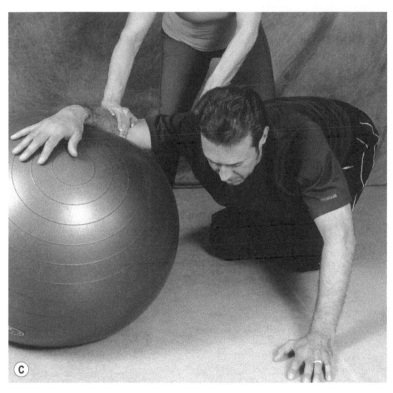

Figure 6.33c
PNF

Practitioner:

- Stand either behind or in front of the client – whichever feels best for you.

- Place one of your hands on the lateral border of their scapula on the joint line.

- Angle your hand in slightly toward the scapula and gently downward.

- Place your other hand on the lateral aspect their elbow and either press it down into the ball or pull it away, but in either case, traction elbow away from shoulder joint.

- Your resistance remains steady – focus on the traction of their arm moving away from their body.

- To increase fibers, roll the ball slightly forward.

- Slowly and gently increase the stretch of their shoulder downward by pressing on scapula.

- Lean away with your body to create traction.

ROM: Retraction of the scapula, drop torso below ball and rotate away from arm on ball.

Traction: Think of creating space between the scapula and their elbow. Traction them away from each other.

PNF:

- Get the client to lift their body up into your hands against your resistance.

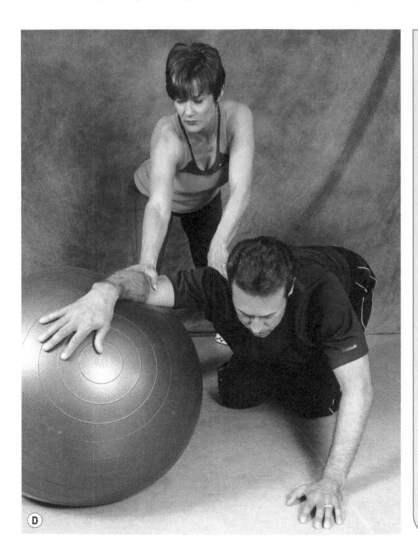

D

Figure 6.33d
Traction

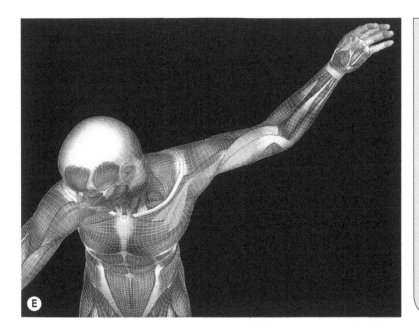

Figure 6.33e
Target tissues primarily within the Deep Front Net

- Get the client to sit back onto both of their hips evenly.

- Get the client to sit back onto the opposite hip from the arm on the ball.

PNF cues:

- "Lift your body up into my hand."

- "Sit back into your hips."

- "Sit back into your opposite hip."

Stretch: Increase retraction of the scapula.

Repeat: PNF two or more times. Play with the angles to target more fibers.

Repeat on the other side.

G. Standing Stretch

1. Standing rhomboids: trunk rotation, shoulder protraction/ flexion – rhomboids – DBAN, SN

Goal: Target tissues lying within the DBAN, SN: rhomboids

Client position:

- Get the client to bend at the waist and hold onto a solid object such as the table.

- Have them stand with their feet hip width apart, knees bent throughout stretch.

- Weight should be evenly distributed over both feet. Watch that they don't shift their weight onto one leg.

- With the arm that's furthest away from you, they reach through and grasp your forearm above the wrist.

Practitioner:

- Turn and face the opposite direction to your client.

- Stand with your feet hip width apart and bend your knees.

- Bend at the waist.

- Place one hand on the underside of their lat and the other grasps their wrist – interlock your wrists for a solid contact.

- Rotate their lat upward toward the ceiling as you pull their arm across their body, rotating their body toward you. The focus is on rotating the torso, not pulling the arm across.

ROM: Trunk rotation.

Traction: Think of rotating their torso away from their arm.

PNF: Get the client to pull their arm and shoulder back across themselves and rotate away from you.

Cue for PNF: "Pull your torso and arm away from me."

Stretch: Increase trunk rotation.

Repeat: PNF two or more times. Play with the angles to target more fibers.

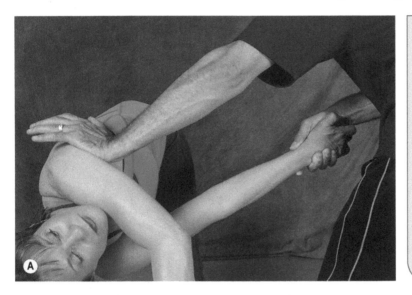

Figure 6.34a
Rhomboids hand placement

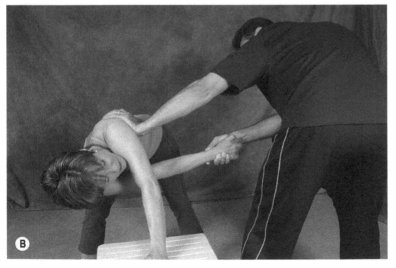

Figure 6.34b
ROM

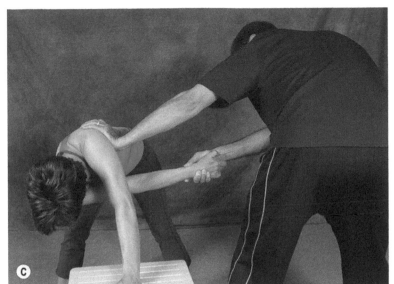

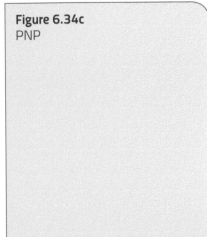

Figure 6.34c
PNP

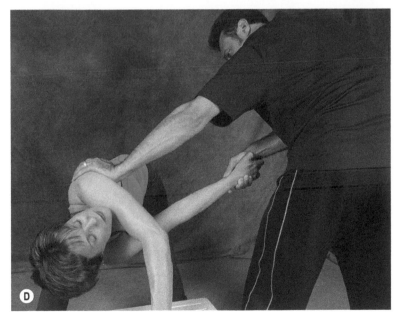

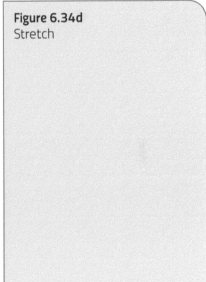

Figure 6.34d
Stretch

ADLs	Activities of Daily Living
AROM	Active Range of Motion
CRAC	Contract-Relax-Antagonist-Contract
DBAN	Deep Back Arm Net
DFAN	Deep Front Arm Net
DFN	Deep Front Net
DOMS	Delayed Onset Muscle Soreness
FN	Functional Net
FST	Fascial Stretch Therapy™
GTO	Golgi Tendon Organ
H-R	Hold-Relax
HVLA	High Velocity Low Amplitude
IR	Internal Rotation
LLD	Leg Length Discrepancy
LN	Lateral Net
MET	Muscle Energy Technique
PMJN	Posture Myofascia Joint Nerve
PNF	Proprioceptive Neuromuscular Facilitation
PNS	Parasympathetic Nervous System
PROM	Passive Range of Motion
PTSD	Post-traumatic Stress Disorder
PRT	Positional Release Technique
R1	Resistance 1
R2	Resistance 2
RROM	Resistive Range of Motion
RT	Resistance to Traction
SITTT	Scan-Identify-Test-Treat-Test again
SBAN	Superficial Back Arm Net
SBN	Superficial Back Net
SFAN	Superficial Front Arm Net
SFN	Superficial Front Net
SIJ	Sacroiliac Joint
SLR	Straight Leg Raising
SN	Spiral Net
SNS	Sympathetic Nervous System
SOAP	Subjective Objective Assessment Plan
SSS	Stretch-Shorten-or-Stabiliz
TOC	Traction Oscillation Circumduction

Note: Page numbers followed by f and b indicates figure and box respectively